Remedies for . . .

*Backache
*Nightmares
*Bronchitis
*Hay Fcvcr
*Heartburn
*Morning sickness

. . . and many other ailments can be found in *Homegrown Healing*—a unique guide to the folk medicine of Mexico. With an A-to-Z index of ailments and specific instructions on preparing remedies using natural ingredients, this book allows anyone to make use of the timeless wisdom passed down from the ancient cultures—and still in use in modern Mexico today.

Homegrown Healing

HOMEGROWN HEALING

Traditional Home Remedies from Mexico

Annette Sandoval

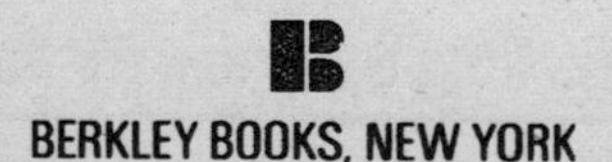

BERKLEY BOOKS, NEW YORK

1-HERBOLOGY
2-MEDICINAL PLANTS

If you purchased this book without a cover, you should be aware that this book is stolen property. It was reported as "unsold and destroyed" to the publisher, and neither the author nor the publisher has received any payment for this "stripped book."

HOMEGROWN HEALING

A Berkley Book / published by arrangement with
the author

PRINTING HISTORY
Berkley edition / March 1998

The Penguin Putnam Inc. World Wide Web site address is
http://www.penguinputnam.com

ISBN: 0-425-16155-2

BERKLEY®
Berkley Books are published by The Berkley Publishing Group,
a member of Penguin Putnam Inc., 200 Madison Avenue,
New York, New York 10016.
BERKLEY and the "B" design are trademarks belonging to
Berkley Publishing Corporation.

PRINTED IN THE UNITED STATES OF AMERICA

10 9 8 7 6 5 4 3 2 1

For my nieces and nephews:

Mia, Marissa, Jordan, Dillon Santiago,
Christopher, and Andrés.

Affirm the past and your
futures will never be denied.

Acknowledgments

Thanks to:

M.E.Ch.A., Lillian Castillo-Speed, for allowing me to utilize the Chicano Studies Library at U.C. Berkeley; the staff at the Strybing H.C.H. Library; Pachita Sandoval and France Sandoval; Marty Sandoval; Richard Chabran; Carmelita La Roche; Miriam Wolf; Mario Araujo; Candelario Barragan and Enedina Barragan; Jose Calderon; Teresa Salazar; Illiana Cantu and the women in her family; Antonio Gallegos Cantu Nava; Guilliemina Gallegos Ferrea; Elisa Gallegos and Rosa Gallegos; Sergio De La Riva and his mom, Maria Elena Rivas De La Riva; Dan Garcia; my angels, Lisa Garcia and her grandmother, Otilia Lugo; Deann Lucky Gallegos and her grandmother, Feliciana ''Bessie'' G. Castillo, for keeping the traditions alive; Trinadad C. Quiroz and Rosalia Moya; Christine Granados and her *abuelita*, Oralia Tellez of El Paso, Texas; Hero; Lilia Hernandez; Leticia Valdez; Gazel Valdez; Lisa Loyo and her grandmother, Emmanuela Loyo; Lourdes Tapia and her mom, Rosa Elva Gonzalez; Arturo Sanchez and his grandma, Ma.de la Luz Aguirre; Jonathan Semer; Mark Anthony Torres and his ancestors from Zacatecas; Dolores Guena-Urquidi and her grandmother, Pachuco; Aaron Vasquez; Jeffrey Michael Villalobos and Feliz Villalobos, his grandmother; Andrea Arguijo Galvan and Elenore Martinez Arguijo; Andrea Vasquez; Jacqueline Olvera and her mother, Cristina Olvera; Joe (Gordo) Sanchez; Ricardo Araiza and his wife, Karina Paredes; Ana Serrato; Mercedes Ja Gaiten-Gonzalez; George Lopez; Jordi Sod Hoffs; Hector Torres, Abbey Phalen; Robert Vazquez; Mireya Almeida and Aurora Quintero; Lucy Chapa; Eliseo Torres; Raymond Guerro; Laura Munoz.

Especially, I thank (God for) you, Patrick Phalen.

Contents

Introduction

De médico, poeta, músico y loco todos tenemos un poco.

Of doctor, poet, musician and madman we each have a trace.

I remember my eldest sister, Yola, waking up in the middle of the night unable to breathe. My mother made a quick dash to the kitchen, and we soon heard chopping and sizzling sounds. My siblings, my father, and I watched in helpless amazement as Yola's puckering face turned bright red, then dark red. Before Yola had a chance to go purple, my mother was at her bedside with a diaper full of steaming aromatic "stuff." She placed the poultice on Yola's neck, and within seconds her breathing and fair complexion had returned. I was convinced that Mother knew magic.

During my childhood trips back to Jalisco, Mexico, I noticed that women often referred to plants as if they were people. Each herb, according to their conversations, maintained its own unique personality. Some herbs are deceptive—stay away from those. Some are very helpful with childbirth or when feeling depressed. Others may not do much, but they sure make for good dinner companions. Even small children were familiar with the herbal ways. While shooting marbles one shadeless afternoon with my younger cousins, I was introduced to the delicate technique of curing a sty with a lemon seed.

Later, my father landed a union job, complete with medical and dental insurance. I guess my mother felt that her *remedios caseros* were inferior to the teamsters' health plan, and promptly shifted from plants to prescriptions. Needless to say, most of the traditional remedies evaporated from my family's cupboards—and memories—soon after.

• • •

Recently, I had been on the lookout for alternative forms of home-based healing. Even with the breakthroughs in modern science, I felt caught in the backlash of progress, and experienced feelings of alienation from our health care system. I missed the holistic approach to healing, the intrinsic kindness of human touch, the impression that warmed herbs left on all of my senses. I decided to reclaim this lost tradition.

On my next trip to the library, I drifted over to the folk remedies section. I was dismayed by the lack of information available on the curative practices of Mexico. The shelves were well stocked with Chinese, Ayurvedic, and American folk medicine—and even a book on Maori healing—but next to nothing from the culture at our proximate border.

After a year and a half of research, I accumulated a number of valuable resources by dedicated ethnobotanists, grandmothers, and even herbal enthusiasts on the Internet. A key contact was M.E.Ch.A (*Movimiento Estudiantil Chicano de Aztlán*), a national organization for Chicano/Mexican students located on high schools and college campuses. I posed the question, "When you were a child and became ill, how would your *abuelita* (grandmother) take care of you?" The response was impressive. It appears that these students and their families enjoyed reliving these memories. I was flooded with letters and e-mail by these individuals who, in turn, learned about their culture and themselves.

Though the details of the cures vary from region to region, there are consistencies throughout Mexican America. For example, I received remedies for potato poultices from several states via e-mail. Although they varied slightly, methods in preparing the potato remedies were almost exact, affirming the successive oral passage of this tradition.

This book is for people who would rather reach into their kitchen cupboard instead of their medicine cabinet for relief. It allows the reader to experience a cultural approach to self-care, while stimulating the imagination with reflections of Mexico's rich folklore and beliefs.

Chapter 1

The Healers of Aztlan

No le pido a Dios que me dé;
nomás que me ponga donde hay.

I never ask God to give me anything;
I only ask him to put me where things are.

Mexican folk medicine is a healing philosophy with several disparate pasts. Two significant influences are the seemingly incompatible races of the American Indian and the Spanish conquistadores. The fusion of these two cultures has created the unique healing philosophy of the Mexican people.

Before the arrival of the Spaniards, Mesoamerica (the area of central Mexico, Belize, Guatemala, and parts of Honduras) had been agricultural for over 3,000 years. A connection between nature, religion, and health was slowly established. The Aztecs referred to this delicate balance as a "harmony" between themselves and nature. Tilting one's balance would cause serious illness or death. Similarly, the Spaniards believed that health was God's will, and could be taken away as rectification.

In the fifteenth century, the Huaxtepec garden was developed by Moctezuma I. It housed a collection of several thousand medicinal plants. Academic priests conducted research with plant derivatives for their pharmacological benefits. About this same time, Spain was leading in European medical advancement. Its superiority in medicine had been due, in part, to the knowledge acquired while under Arabic rule.

In the sixteenth century, the Spanish conquistadores first set foot in the New World. The ancient codices of the Aztec priests were considered blasphemous by Catholic priests, prompting Hernán Cortés to order all works on botany and science to be destroyed. The values, convictions, and traditions of the Aztec people were almost completely eradicated by Spain in a relatively short period of time.

The early missionaries played a paradoxical role in salvaging the remnants of Aztec knowledge. They traveled throughout *Nuevo España* collecting and documenting *materia médica,* while integrating European healing philosophies. The friars also introduced the Catholic faith and prayers to saints for curing illnesses. Some of the native remedies have survived the conquest due to quick-thinking native healers who renamed the plants used in ancient ceremonial practices, using the names of benevolent saints.

The Spaniards introduced *humoral pathology*—Hippocrates' theory that health depends on the proper distribution of the body's four humors: blood, phlegm, yellow bile, and black bile. From humoral pathology, the hot-and-cold theory of disease has survived in Mexico and in the southwestern United States. In order to restore the body's symmetry, people who subscribe to this theory take plants with opposing qualities.

From the sixteenth to the nineteenth centuries, a great quantity of the Americas' medicinal plants and vegetation, such as potatoes and corn, were shipped to Europe. Likewise, Old World plants such as chamomile and lemons were imported to the Americas. Medieval superstitions, including witchcraft and sorcery, were also introduced to Mesoamerica by the conquerors.

Fortunately, many remedies survived the conquest and are still used in Mexican America. The Mexican Institute for the Study of Medical Plants was established in 1975. Researchers at the institute have been examining the sixteenth-century records to determine the validity of indigenous medicines, with great success. Science, which had dismissed traditional remedies, has begun to reevaluate the therapeutic values of botanical lore.

Today, folk medicine and modern science maintain a symbiotic relationship within the Mexican and Chicano communities. Traditional Mexican healing subscribes to the belief that some physical ailments may be caused by supernatural or social causes, while allopathic medicine's approach to illness, until recently, has been strictly biochemical. Both practices are respected and are considered by some to be different branches of the same healing tree. Many choose to utilize both methods of treatment at the same time.

For centuries, folk remedies have been preserved and administered by the women of the household. These remedies have been passed down not only from mothers to daughters, but across the backyard fence and at social gatherings. When a family member becomes ill, mothers rely on these remedies and treatments.

Much of the population is still devoted to the curative practice of *curanderismo*, or "folk healing." A *yerbera* (herbalist), a *sobadora* (massage therapist), or a *partera* (midwife) may be called upon to cure ailments of the body and, just as important, the soul. Unlike allopathic medicine, these practices connect, even overlap. If a condition persists, a *curandera*, or healer, may be called in. The *curandera* is usually contacted after some or all of these resources have been exhausted.

Yerberas focus on administering herbal remedies and proper diet. Comparable to botanists, they are also well versed in the cycles of plants and the harvesting periods. A *yerbera* (or her male equivalent, the *yerbero*) can identify hundreds of species of plants, along with their therapeutic properties and means of prescription. She believes that nature has provided us with a cure for every disease.

The *sobadora* is responsible for the treatment of sprains

and broken bones. Knowledgeable in acupressure, the *sobadora* (or *sobador*) alleviates stomach conditions such as *empacho* (the belief that food has lodged in the digestive tract) and gives general massage therapy.

The practice of the *partera* includes prenatal care, childbirth, postpartum care, and pediatrics. Midwifery is the only field to be recognized by allopathic medicine, and is experiencing an upsurge of interest by women choosing to participate in the childbirth process. This less expensive option is a valued resource for Mexican and Chicana women.

The *curandera* (or *curandero*) is the most revered of the healers. She blends a complex system of religion, rituals, and herbs to treat the infirm, and is responsible for maintaining the emotional, cultural, and health requirements within the community. She is an authority on folk illnesses such as *susto* (fright sickness), a malady that allopathic medicine has dismissed as groundless.

Many *curanderas* believe that they were chosen by God to do His work. This is referred to as *el don*, or "the gift." The *curandera* usually begins her apprenticeship by curing family members and neighbors, under the watchful eye of an elder *curandera*. Through word of mouth, a successful *curandera*'s circle widens. Her techniques and reputation in caring for the community may spread throughout the region, occasionally becoming legendary. Some *curanderas* are said to apply the laying of hands to cure physical and emotional illness.

The word *curandera* derives from the verb *curar*, meaning "to heal." A *curandera's* job, through God's will, is to realign the body and soul. In the healing process, the patient's social, physical, and emotional states are taken into consideration before a diagnosis is determined. Treatments vary according to the patient's condition and the *curandera's* knowledge.

The *curandera* often begins by talking to the patient's family, creating an intense bond among all of the parties. Her patients vary from those trying to ease the pain of an incurable disease to those seeking help in deflecting a curse from a jealous neighbor. The *curandera* may petition *espiritos* (spirits); utilize symbolic objects such as candles, eggs, and holy water; or dispense herbs. If the patient does not improve, this too is God's will.

Religion and the supernatural are linked within the Mexican community. Some believe that illness is natural, a punishment, or one's destiny. Superstitions serve to uphold the culture's convictions by enforcing predetermined values and traditions onto the individual. They also provide an explanation for the unknown. Falling off a ladder, for example, may be the result of treating others poorly or missing mass.

Once cured, the patient will usually compensate the *curandera* through a gift of food, livestock, or a monetary donation. Prayers and pilgrimages to shrines of the benevolent saints of the disorder may be required by the recovered.

For many Mexicans, choosing between a healer and a physician depends on a number of factors. Some of the more immediate considerations are the seriousness of the condition, the expense of treatment, and the accessibility of a clinic. Other factors include how traditional the patient is, the *curandera*'s knowledge of the illness, and of course, the patient's faith.

Chapter 2

The Kitchen Clinic

Nadie sabe lo que contiene la olla,
nomás la cucharra que la menea.

No one knows what is in the pot,
except the spoon that stirs the contents.

Most kitchen cupboards are already well stocked with remedies for many of our common ailments. Potatoes, garlic, and pinto beans might be part of tonight's dinner, but they also work wonders on insect bites, weak fingernails, and canker sores; those jars of oregano, thyme, and cinnamon can go a long way in helping indigestion, asthma, and nausea.

However, some of the cures in this book contain less common ingredients, indigenous to Mexico, but not likely to be found in many local supermarkets. Most herbs are available at health food stores, or you can order them by mail from the sources listed in Chapter 5. I've also included treatments that use rather exotic ingredients. You may not want to use spiderwebs, donkey milk, or horse saliva, and I think you may have difficulty finding some of these items. I've presented these folk remedies to illustrate the wide variety of cures and the rich, deeply rooted tradition of Mexican healing. Finally, I do not condone the slaughtering of young hens (see "Lung Conditions," Chapter 3); I would simply like you to know that this was a common folk cure that is rarely used today.

In the following pages, you will find a list of common

ailments and Mexican home remedies to treat them. They have been tested throughout the years and have been passed down from generation to generation. I cannot say from personal experience that they all work, nor should they be a substitute for seeing your doctor when necessary. Use this book as a reference guide, find the treatments that work for you, and pass them along to your *nietos* (grandchildren).

Many of the treatments in this book contain herbs that you probably have in your kitchen. However, though dried herbs maintain their flavor, they do lose some of their medicinal potency in a relatively short period of time. Consider purchasing herbs at health food stores or from retail catalogs (see Chapter 5). Whenever possible, grow your own herbs. This will not only ensure freshness, but it will also allow you to pick the herbs at the height of their potency.

General Rules to Follow When Using Herbs

THOUGH HERBS ARE efficacious for general ailments, they can do only so much. Like over-the-counter medicines, excessive use or misuse of herbs may be harmful. Before utilizing the remedies in chapter 3, "Homegrown Wisdom," refer to the warnings on the medicinal usage of herbs in chapter 4, "Remedies at a Glance." If a patient experiences any type of side effects, rashes, or the like, stop home treatment. Always consult a physician before treatment. If the condition has not improved in two weeks, consult your physician. Above all else, use common sense.

INFANTS, CHILDREN, AND SENIOR CITIZENS:

Always consult a physician before administering remedies to children, infants, or senior citizens. Never give herbs to infants under a year old without consulting a physician. When administering herbs to children and seniors, use a half or a quarter dose. If medicine is not palatable, sweeten it with sugar. Never give honey to young children; some honey is highly toxic, and may be fatal.

PREGNANCY:

Women in their first trimester of pregnancy should not take any type of medication, including herbs. Pregnant women in their second or third trimester of pregnancy should always consult a physician before taking herbal medication.

PHARMACEUTICAL PRESCRIPTIONS:

Consult with your physician before combining herbal medication with prescription or over-the-counter drugs. Many prescription medications contain plant derivatives; the patient may be in danger of over-medication.

PREPARATION OF HERBS

PREPARATION AND APPLICATION of herbal remedies is just as important as the ingredients. Glass, earthenware, or stainless steel mixing bowls are recommended. Always avoid using aluminum, iron, or plastic receptacles. The following guidelines are suggestions in preparing internal and external botanicals in order to maximize their healing benefits.

TEAS

THE MAJORITY OF remedies listed in this book are as easy to make as a cup of tea. There are two methods for preparing teas: decoctions and infusions. The standard dose for teas is 1 teaspoon dry herbs or 2 teaspoons fresh herbs per cup of water. Teas lose their therapeutic properties relatively quickly. A fresh batch should be made every day. When administering teas to children and senior citizens, cut the dose to a half or a quarter.

DECOCTIONS:

The *decoction* method extracts the medicinal properties from tough substances such as bark and rhizomes. The standard dosage for a decoction is 1 teaspoon dried and crushed (or powdered) herbs or 2 teaspoons freshly chopped and crushed herbs per cup of water. To make a decoction, put the plant material in cold water, then cover and bring to a boil. Reduce heat and simmer for 30 minutes to an hour. Strain the decoction and sip ½ cup three times a day.

INFUSIONS:

An *infusion* is used to separate the volatile oils that are found in the soft parts of the plant, such as the leaves, flowers, and stems. To make an infusion, boil water, then remove it from the heat source. Pour a splash of the hot water into the teapot, swirl it around, then rinse. Place the herbs in the clean teapot. Since bubbling water may cause medicinal properties to evaporate, wait for the remaining water to be still before pouring it over the herbs. Cover the teapot, and let the tea steep for at least 10 minutes. The longer it steeps, the stronger the infusion becomes. Strain the tea and drink ½ cup three times a day, or as instructed.

TINCTURES

A TINCTURE IS an herbal extraction with an alcohol-and-water base. The alcohol not only breaks up the active ingredients of the herb, but preserves them as well. If stored in a dark, cool place, tinctures have a shelf life of up to two years. In health food stores, tinctures may be prepared with ethyl alcohol, but for home use, grain alcohol of at least 60 proof should be used. Never take rubbing alcohol (isopropyl alcohol) internally; it is extremely toxic.

To make a tincture, select just one herb. Finely chop and bruise the plant and place it in a large glass container. Pour 3 parts alcohol, vodka, or grain alcohol and 2 parts water over 1 part herb, then seal the jar. Store in a dark place for two weeks, shaking every other day. Press and strain mixture, then pour it into a sterilized bottle. Take ½ teaspoon of the tincture twice a day. To make a tincture palatable, add honey or stir it into a cup of water with fruit juice. To dissipate most of the alcohol, pour the tincture into hot water, then drink it when it is cool.

COMPRESSES

A *COMPRESS* IS used to treat skin and muscle injuries. Soak a clean cotton cloth in a hot or cold infusion, decoction, or tincture, then apply it to the affected area.

OILS

THE METHOD FOR making *massage oil* is similar to that for making a tincture; oil is substituted for the alcohol and water.

OINTMENTS/SALVES

AN *OINTMENT* FORMS a protective covering on the skin. In Mexican households, ointments are traditionally made with lard or oil and herbs, but petroleum jelly or vegetable shortening are often substituted.

The following is a quick and simple way to make an ointment: In a double boiler, heat ½ to 1 cup lard or petroleum jelly until melted. Add 2 tablespoons fresh, finely chopped herbs, then heat for 30 minutes to one hour. Strain then store the mixture in a jar. Use when needed. The ointment could have a shelf life of up to one year.

POULTICES

A *POULTICE* IS applied much like a compress. Instead of herbal extracts, a layer of plant material is applied to the skin. To prepare a poultice, finely chop fresh or dried herbs and place them in a bowl. Pour a small amount of hot water or oil over the herbs, just enough to make the mixture into a mash. Rub oil on the skin, to keep herbs from sticking. Apply the hot or cold poultice to the affected area, then cover it with gauze. A poultice can also be put between layers of cotton or gauze and applied to the affected area. Change the poultice every few hours, or as needed.

Chapter 3

Homegrown Wisdom

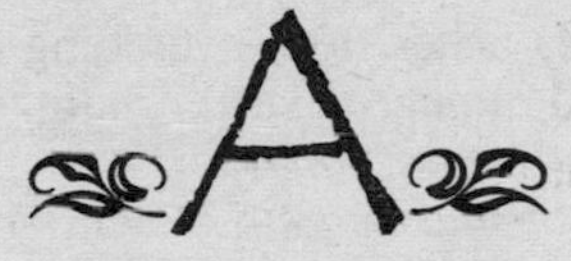

Quien quiera al arbol
tiene que querer a sus ramas.

He who cares for the
tree must also care for the branches

Abscesses

Split open a *maguey* (century plant) leaf, releasing a gel. Heat the gel until it is warm and apply to the abscess.

Mix 2 tablespoons chopped *toloache* (jimson weed) with ½ cup of melted *manteca* (lard). Heat mixture for 30 minutes. Cool ointment and place directly on the abscess. You should feel relief right away.

Mix a handful of crushed *llantén* (plantain) weed and enough *manteca* to act as a binder. If *manteca* is not available, try shortening. Apply this poultice on the abscess until swelling and pain are gone.

ACHES

Massage sore muscles with a tincture or salve made with arnica flowers. This will reduce the pain and bring down any swelling.

For sore muscles, rub an *aguacate* (avocado) pit tincture on the aches.

When your body aches from overdoing it, try an *alcanfor* (camphor) and *manteca* (lard) rubdown.

Rub a tincture of *uña de gato* (catclaw) on the sore muscles.

If an ache is centered in one place, combine chopped *toloache* (jimson weed) and heated lard. Apply the poultice to the sore area, then cover.

Combine *yerba buena* (mint) with melted lard or petroleum jelly. Rub ointment on aching muscles.

Mix white dry mustard and enough tequila to make a paste. Place the mixture in the sun, until warm, then apply to the lower back. Cover with a warm towel.

ACNE

Wash face, then rinse with a *flor saúco* (elder flowers) infusion.

To cure acne, eat two cloves of raw *ajo* (garlic) a day, one in the morning and the other at night. Continue for a month, and the acne will be cured.

Afterbirth

Malva (mallow) tea boiled with raisins will expel the afterbirth from the mother's body.

Air Freshener

To keep closets from getting musty during the season of heavy rains, hang some *alfafón* (sweet clover).

Aire (the cold)

Aire *is a condition caused by going from one extreme temperature to another. An example of this would be running, then taking a cold shower. There are two different types of* aire. *The first occurs in children, affecting the ears. The second befalls adults, and may lead to facial paralysis and muscular spasms.*

Carry the root of the *oshá* (lovage) plant in your pocket for protection against *aire*.

When *aire* gets in you, and sits like a cold bubble in your head, burn *ruda* (rue) on hot coals and inhale the smoke. That night, sleep on a pillow stuffed with dry *ruda*. The *aire* will seep out while you sleep.

If the unwelcome chill settles in the stomach, drink any of the following infusions with honey before going to bed:

***Canela* (cinnamon bark) tea**
***Cilantro* (coriander) seeds tea**
***Epazote* (wormseed) tea**
***Romero* (rosemary) tea**
***Ruda* (rue) tea**

Allergies

See Hay Fever

Amoebas

The best quick cure for ridding the body of amoebas or intestinal parasites is by eating plenty of guavas. Eat three before breakfast, then two before lunch, and one before dinner. Patients are usually cured of diarrhea and cramps before they tire of the fruit.

Anemia

If you suffer from anemia, drink a tea made with dry alfalfa seeds throughout the day.

To thicken the blood, drink *cola de caballo* (horsetail) tea.

Aphrodisiac

When your spouse begins to lose interest in the bedroom, a few drops of damiana tincture will keep the blankets tangled.

Drink ½ cup of *Raíz del Macho* (muira puama) tea first thing in the morning until desired results are obtained. This should take less than a week.

Zarzaparrilla (sarsaparilla) root tea is said to intensify sexual desire.

Appetite Stimulant

It is said that hunger is the best spice for food. The following decoctions have played a part in great meals for centuries. The appetite will improve if the teas are drunk every morning, on an empty stomach:

***Albahaca* (basil) tea**

Alfalfa tea

***Anís de estrella* (star anise) tea**

***Hinojo* (fennel) seed tea**

Laurel tea

***Marrubio* (Horehound) tea**

To elicit hunger, chew slowly on just one *sabino* (juniper) berry.

Drink a cold tea of *cuasia* (quassia). This will stimulate hunger. Some say it remedies the problem of anorexia.

Appetite Suppressant

Yerba maté tea will help curb the appetite.

Arthritis

For inflammation of the joints that results in pain and swelling, sip on a tea made with *fresno* (ash) leaves, *cola de caballo* (horsetail), or *jarita* (willow bark).

Mash then strain enough gel from the aloe vera plant to make 1 teaspoon aloe vera juice. Add liquid to a glass of orange juice or water, and drink every morning before breakfast.

For quick relief throughout the day, peel off the outer layer of the aloe vera leaf, then heat the gel. Apply to the affected area while still hot, as hot as you can stand it. Carefully wrap with clean rags or gauze.

Soak the affected area in a basin of hot water and aloe vera extract.

Rub a tequila and *fresno* (ash) leaf tincture on the sore joints.

Spread a poultice of dried *hediondilla* (chaparral) leaves and hot *manteca* (lard) on the painful areas, then wrap.

Simmer dried *hediondilla* (chaparral) leaves for 10 minutes, strain, then add to bathwater.

Dry and grind *punche* (Indian tobacco), mix with lard, then rub where needed.

Add a handful of crushed *toloache* (jimson weed) leaves to a warm bath and soak yourself. Add a little peyote if you have any around.

Make a tincture with alcohol and minced dried peyote. Place the liquid in a dark cupboard for a couple of weeks. Rub the solution onto the affected area.

Boil a dried *girasol* (sunflower) in a pot of water, then add to a warm bath. Soak until the pain is eased. After your bath, rub a tincture of *girasol* where needed.

Soak in a tub infused with *yerba mansa* (lizard tail) leaves.

ASTHMA

My great-aunt Rosalia Moya told me that during the great epidemic of the early 1900s, a drop of kerosene oil saved her life. She was unable to breathe and her mother put a drop on her tongue, and she was instantly able to inhale. I think kerosene was used often at that time. There weren't many doctors around. My great-uncle Ambrosio Sanchez said that his mother was a doctor. I was impressed. He laughed when I asked him what medical school she went to. He said All mothers were doctors in those days; she either cured you or you died. Life and death were in a delicate balance.

—Dee Gallegos

Inhale the vapors of steamed *eucalipto* (eucalyptus) leaves. You can also burn the mature leaves, then inhale the smoke.

Simmer *marrubio* (horehound) leaves in water and honey until liquid is thick. Take 1 tablespoon every few hours.

Burn dried *punche* (Indian tobacco) and inhale the smoke.

Inhale smoke of *toloache* (jimson weed) to alleviate asthma.

Drink *alhucema* (lavender) and honey tea and place a warm poultice of *alhucema* on the chest.

Mix 1 teaspoon of the powdered root of the *oshá* (lovage) plant into a cup of hot water. Sip slowly.

Drink *cañutillo* (Mormon tea) slowly, so that you inhale the vapors.

Make a tea and a poultice from the leaves and flowers of the *gordolobo* (mullein) plant. Drink from the cup and place the poultice on the chest. The tea leaves will relax the chest, allowing for comfortable breathing. An alternative to this method is to burn and inhale *gordolobo* smoke.

Take 1 tablespoon honey with minced *tomillo* (thyme) until symptoms are gone.

Sip *yerba santa* (mountain balm) tea.

Athlete's Foot

Before going to bed, wash feet, then pat dry. Peel off the outer layer of the aloe vera leaf and heat the gel. Apply the gel to the affected area while it is still hot, as hot as you can stand it. Carefully cover feet with cotton socks, rags, or gauze. Continue to do this every night, even for an additional three nights after the itching stops. During the daylight hours, avoid shoes that don't breathe. If possible, go barefoot. If you live by the beach, walk in the hot sand; fungus hates that.

To stop fungal infection, soak your feet in a hot infusion of *llantén* (plantain) leaf. During the day, alleviate itching by placing bruised *llantén* leaves in your shoes.

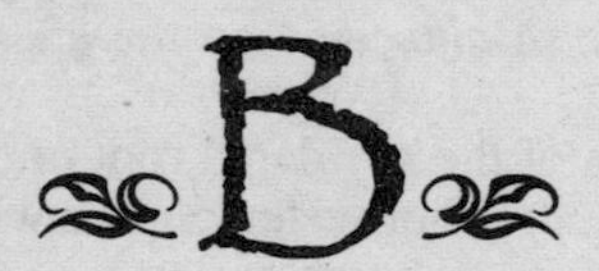

Un hombre sin alegría no es bueno o no está bueno.

A man without happiness is either not good or not well.

Backache

For discomfort or pain, make a hot poultice of *siempreviva* (stonecrop) and apply to the back or spine area. Change every few hours.

Place a coin directly on the affected area of the back. Put a lit candle directly on the coin. Cover the candle with a small glass container. You will notice that as soon as the flame goes out, the skin begins to extend. Do not be alarmed; it's just the *aire* being pulled out from under the skin. You can now slide the glass over the surface of the back to pull the remaining *aire* out. After the cupping, massage olive oil on the back.

Bee Stings

Apply cooked *col* (cabbage) at room temperature directly on the bee sting, then wrap with clean gauze or rags.

Dab honey from the hive on a sting.

Bilis

Bilis is an illness resulting from an increase of bile in the system. This is the result of repressed anger, creating a bad disposition. The symptoms include gas and constipation. The patient is usually encouraged to express his or her feelings and drink herbal teas.

When you are suffering from *bilis,* drink one of the following teas:

Canela **(cinnamon bark) and honey tea**

Estafiate **(wormwood) tea**

Flor saúco **(elder flowers) tea**

Oshá **(lovage) root tea**

Simmer 2 teaspoons dry or 4 teaspoons fresh *cabellos de elote* (corn silk) with 2 cups water until the water turns dark brown, then sip the entire mixture.

Birth Control

See Contraception

Bladder Infections

For bladder infections, drink a tea made of *jarita* (willow bark).

Blood Pressure

To level your blood pressure, drink alfalfa tea every morning.

Sip on a *flor saúco* (elder flowers) infusion.

To bring blood pressure down, bathe in a tub of warm water mixed with a decoction of the young branches of *hediondilla* (chaparral).

If blood pressure tends to run on the high side, eat a raw *ajo* (garlic) clove in the morning with a glass of milk or water, then again at night before going to bed.

Fresh *perejil* (parsley) tea helps maintain blood pressure.

Blood Tonic

An excellent blood purifier is made by tossing some fresh *chicória* (dandelion) leaves into a salad. Eat every now and again to thin your blood of poisons.

Sasafrás (sassafras) tea taken every morning makes a good blood tonic.

When your blood is sick, boil *zarzaparrilla* (sarsaparilla) root, then drink the tea.

Boils

To take care of a small boil, make *masa* (cornmeal). Instead of forming a tamale, spread it in the center of a long strip of cloth and wrap it around the boil while still hot. The next day, the core of the boil can easily be removed.

When a boil just sits there and refuses to go away, place *toloache* (jimson weed) heated with melted lard directly on the boil, then wrap into place. This will prompt it to pop.

Bruise the leaves of the *llantén* (plantain) weed, apply to the boil, then cover with a clean cloth. Change daily.

Bone Cancer

To reduce the pains brought on by bone cancer, apply a marijuana poultice on the affected area, then wrap with gauze or rags.

Breasts (sore)

When breasts are sore and tender, apply an *alfafón* (sweet clover) poultice.

Broken Bones

To help mend a crack or rupture in bone or cartilage, there is nothing better than a poultice of *consuelda* (comfrey) root. Just apply to the surface of the affected area, then wrap the poultice into place with gauze or clean rags.

Set the broken bone, then apply a poultice made from the root of the *oshá* (lovage) plant and *punche* (Indian tobacco).

BRONCHITIS

To ease the congestion brought on by bronchitis, take an angélica tincture in a cup of water or juice. This will also help bring up the phlegm.

For bronchial infection accompanied by fever, drink *borraja* (borage) tea.

A decoction made from *clavos* (cloves) will bring up the phlegm.

First, apply a poultice of *consuelda* (comfrey) on the chest. Then drink a decoction of *consuelda* root. Inhale the vapors and sip the liquid.

Inhale fresh *eucalipto* (eucalyptus) steam to soothe bronchial infection.

Simmer two *ajo* (garlic) bulbs in 1 cup water until liquid is reduced by half. Pour into a bowl, then mash ½ cup sugar into bowl until the consistency thickens. Take 1 tablespoon three times a day.

Simmer *marrubio* (horehound) leaves and honey until mixture thickens. Take 1 tablespoon every few hours.

When the chest feels tight like a drum, make a tea and a poultice from *gordolobo* (mullein) leaves and stems. The poultice will relax the chest, and the tea will allow for comfortable breathing.

For bronchitis and phlegm buildup, try oregano tea.

Take a *tomillo* (thyme) tincture two or three times a day.

Drink *yerba santa* (mountain balm) tea. Apply a poultice of *yerba santa* and lard to the chest.

BRUISES

Rub a tincture of aloe vera and alcohol onto the bruise. It will be gone in half of the time that it would usually take to fade.

Rub bruise with a tincture or salve made from dried arnica flowers. This will fade the colors and bring down any swelling.

For discoloration of the skin, rub a tincture of *uña de gato* (catclaw) onto the bruise.

A good ointment for bruises is *consuelda* (comfrey) with lard.

Rub menthol on injuries so that they won't bruise. It works!

When your bruise looks more like an eggplant than skin, apply a *pasionaria* (passionflower) poultice.

A poultice of *yerba mansa* (lizard tail) root speeds the healing of bruises.

BUMPS

Rub vinegar and salt on the bump.

Burning Urination

Simmer 1 teaspoon dry or 2 teaspoons fresh *cabellos de elote* (corn silk) with 1 cup water until the water turns dark brown. The tea will flush out the burning feeling when you urinate.

Burns

Whenever someone gets burned, wash the affected area thoroughly. Break off a piece of the lower leaf of the aloe vera plant and apply the fresh gel directly onto the burn.

A good way to cool a burn when you are cooking is to smear a cooked *fríjol* (bean) on the burn. Of course, the *fríjol* should be at room temperature in order for this to work.

A raw egg will cool a burn quickly, and will help prevent blistering and scarring.

Dab some honey on a burn to keep it from getting infected.

Coat a burn with lard. This will seal the infection out.

Cover the burn with a minced raw *cebolla* (onion), then wrap it with a clean cloth. Not only will the onion alleviate the pain, but it will prevent the burn from blistering.

For minor burns while cooking, squeeze fresh *juego de naranja* (orange juice) on the burn.

Combine *trementina de piñon* (pine pitch) and lard over low heat. Once the mixture turns into a liquid, remove from heat, strain, and apply to the burn. The ointment will keep for several months.

Smudge some *barro* (mud) on the burn.

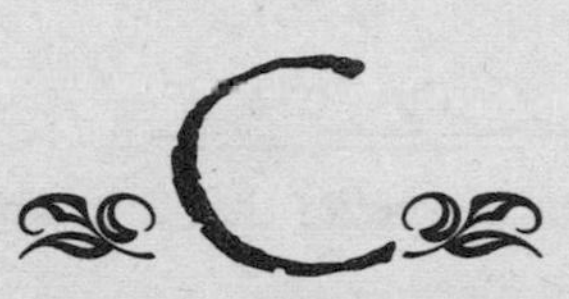

Cada quien se rasca con sus uñas.

Each one should scratch himself with his own fingernails.

Caída de la Mollera

Caída de la mollera, *or depressed fontanel, is a syndrome that occurs only with infants. It is believed to be caused by pulling a nursing baby from the mother's nipple too abruptly, when the infant suckles too greedily, or by a fall from the crib. The symptoms are restlessness, diarrhea, and vomiting, followed by severe dehydration. Physically, the infant appears to wither and the soft spot on the baby's head appears sunken in. This may actually be caused by a viral or bacterial infection. Immediate medical attention is recommended.*

A common remedy is to coat the thumb with salt, then place against the child's palate. This will push the fontanel back up.

Calcium Deficiency

In a bowl, mix a pulverized eggshell with lemon juice. Leave the mixture out that night. You'll notice that the shell has dissolved. Drink the mixture in the morning. This is a perfect way for pregnant women to absorb calcium quickly.

Calluses

Paint calluses with red nail polish and they will fall off.

Cancer (deterrent)

It has long been the belief that a lemon a day keeps the cancer away.

Canker Sores

The next time you get a puffy *grano* (canker sore) in your mouth, cut an uncooked pinto bean in half lengthwise and place it directly on the sore. For some reason, the bean dries up the *grano* and makes it stop stinging. However, it may sting when the bean is first placed on it.

Carsickness

Here is a really simple remedy to keep the kids from experiencing car sickness: let them suck on one piece of cinnamon or ginger candy all the way through the trip. If that sounds like too much sugar for your children, consider the alternative.

Chest Colds

Dry and grind *punche* (Indian tobacco), mix with lard, then rub on the chest.

Mix 1 teaspoon of powdered root from the *oshá* (lovage) plant into a cup of hot water, then add a little whiskey and honey. This will get the patient to sweat out the impurities and will rid the chest of phlegm.

Chest Infection

Place a poultice of *cola de caballo* (horsetail) stalks on the chest.

Chicken Pox

Bathe the child in a tub of warm water and *carbonato* (baking soda). Once out of the tub, apply a paste of *carbonato* mixed with a little water.

An *alcanfor* (camphor), *manteca* (lard), and *carbonato* (baking soda) ointment should be dabbed on the skin eruptions. This will keep the child from itching.

A *flor saúco* (elder flowers) tea will ensure that the chicken pox will grow outward instead of inward.

Circulation

To improve your circulation, drink alfalfa tea with a squeeze of lime.

Cirrhosis

In the evening when you have settled in, sip on a tea made with the leaves of the *alcachofa* (artichoke) plant. Then make a poultice from the tea leaves and place it against the liver.

Cocos (Boo-Boos)

When a child gets a scratch or a cut, recite the following chant (while making the sign of the cross on the hurt area):

Sana, Sana	*Heal, heal*
colita de rana	*little frog's tail*
si no sanas hoy	*If you don't recover today*
sanaras	*You will recover*
manana	*tomorrow*

Give the *coco* a kiss, and send the child back out to play.

Colds

Teas for colds should be sipped slowly, so that you inhale the volatile oils escaping in the vapors. Listed here are some suggestions for relieving a cold. Honey and lemon are always welcome accompaniments. Mix your own blend:

Anís **(aniseed) tea**

Canela **(cinnamon bark) tea**

Chile **(cayenne pepper) and lemon tea**

Eucalipto **(eucalyptus) tea**

Hot lemon tea

Laurel tea

Manzanilla **(chamomile), lemon, and honey tea**

Plumajillo **(yarrow) tea**

Romero **(rosemary) tea**

Yerba buena **(mint) tea**

Yerba mansa **(lizard tail) tea**

Yerba santa **(mountain balm) tea**

When you come down with a cold, wait two days before taking a shower. On the third day take a shower, then have someone give you an alcohol rubdown. This will make you drowsy, so you should get under the covers and go to sleep. The next day the cold will be gone.

Suck on half a lime to clear your stuffy nose.

At the onset of a cold, put 4 to 6 prunes, 2 to 3 whole cinnamon sticks, and 2 cups of milk in a pot. Heat the milk until it almost boils, then reduce heat and let the mixture sit for 5 minutes. Take away the cinnamon sticks, then pour the decoction into a mug. Add 1 jigger of brandy and drink hot. Just when you are getting ready to sleep, eat the prunes.

Colic

The following teas will soothe the pain brought on by colic and help the baby to sleep. As a rule, an infant's portion is about ¼ of the adult dosage. Since honey contains tetanus spores, which are dangerous or even fatal to infants and small children, I strongly recommend that you sweeten the tea with sugar instead.

***Aguacate* (avocado) leaves tea**

***Albahaca* (basil) leaves tea**

***Alhucema* (lavender) tea**

***Angélica* tea**

***Anís de estrella* (star anise) tea**

***Flor saúco* (elder flowers) tea**

***Manzanilla* (chamomile) tea**

***Marrubio* (horehound) leaves tea**

***Ruda* (rue) tea**

***Yerba mansa* (lizard tail) leaves tea**

Give the child a weak decoction of *hinojo* (fennel) seeds simmered in milk.

Rosa de Castilla (rose) petals steeped in hot water for a couple of minutes will ease the child's pain.

Congestion

Inhale *alcanfor* (camphor) steam.

Inhale the vapors of *manzanilla* (chamomile) flowers.

Constipation

For difficult, incomplete, or infrequent bowel movement, try one of the following teas:

***Llantén* (plantain) leaf tea**

***Rosa de Castilla* (rose) petals tea**

***Té de sena* (senna tea)**

Prepare *cáscara sagrada* root tea, *al sereno* (make the tea, then let it sit out to catch the night dew) before going to bed. Drink a cup. It usually takes about eight hours to kick in.

Drink a teaspoon of *maguey* (century plant) juice in water.

Chicória (dandelion) leaves, either fresh or in a warm tea, will keep you regular.

Take 1 teaspoon of *grano de lino* (flaxseed), then drink a lot of water.

Mash, then strain enough gel from the aloe vera plant to make 1 teaspoon aloe vera juice. Add the liquid to a glass of orange juice or water.

CONTRACEPTION

In the springtime, chop and crush an entire fresh *flor de Santa Rita* (Indian paintbrush) plant, roots and all. Simmer 1 part plant and 5 parts water. When the liquid has reduced by half, the couple must each drink of it for two weeks. A fresh brew must be made every day. They say this contraception should last six months.

Try douching with a cool infusion of *romero* (rosemary) after being intimate with your husband.

CORAJE

Coraje *is a syndrome entailing uncontrollable fits of rage. Once calmed down, the individual is cured by talking about the fits while drinking tea.*

Simmer *marrubio* (horehound) leaves and honey.

Drink a cold tea of *cuasia* (quassia).

CORNS

Crush a raw *ajo* (garlic) clove, then apply to the corn. Cover with a large bandage.

Paint the corn with red nail polish, and the thickened skin will fall off.

Grind fresh *siempreviva* (stonecrop) leaves with a mortar and pestle, then apply to the corn.

COUGHS

When a child has a cough or there is a buildup of phlegm, make a weak tea of *anís* (aniseed).

Simmer 1 tablespoon *marrubio* (horehound) leaves, 1 tablespoon *oshá* (lovage) and honey with 1 cup water until liquid is left thick. Take 1 tablespoon every few hours.

A very soothing remedy for your children's coughs is to mix *alhucema* (lavender) tea with a teaspoon or two of maple syrup. Kids love it. You may never use store-bought cough syrup again.

Mix 1 teaspoon of the powdered root of the *oshá* (lovage) plant into 1 cup hot water. Add a little whiskey and honey.

For dry hacking coughs, drink a strong tea of *culantrillo* (maidenhair fern) with lots of honey.

A *gordolobo* (mullein) leaves tincture will calm the cough.

Slice a *cebolla morada* (purple onion) into thin spirals and layer. Drizzle them with honey, then place in an airtight container. In three hours, you will notice that the onions have released their sweat. Take 2 tablespoons of this liquid every few hours or as needed to ease the cough.

Sip a *yerba santa* (mountain balm) and honey tea.

Cramps

Place a warm, damp poultice of *alhucemo* (lavender) and *manzanilla* (chamomile) on the abdomen. Then sip on *manzanilla* and honey tea, or take 15 drops of a *manzanilla* tincture.

The following teas also help to ease cramps:

Fresh *perejil* (parsley) tea

***Oshá* (lovage) tea**

***Té de azahar* (orange blossom tea)**

***Yerba buena* (mint) tea**

Sip on a decoction of *clavos* (cloves).

Simmer *cilantro* (coriander) seeds, then drink the tea until the cramps are gone.

Drink a decoction of *hinojo* (fennel) seeds.

Apply a poultice made from the root of the *oshá* (lovage) plant and *punche* (Indian tobacco) to the abdomen.

Make an infusion of *flor de tila* (linden flowers), strain, then add to bathwater.

A tea of *siempreviva* (stonecrop) and *canela* (cinnamon) left out to catch the morning dew will alleviate intestinal cramps.

Place a poultice of grilled *cebolla* (onion) on the abdomen.

Cuts

When a paper cut occurs, apply fresh aloe vera gel directly to the injury.

It is said that if you scrape the mold from old bread or old tortillas, then scatter it on a clean cut, the cut will heal without infection. Do not use rye bread for this; the fungus it produces is highly toxic.

Before you put a bandage on a cut, mash a raw *ajo* (garlic) clove, then put some on the cut.

To keep a cut from getting infected and to promote healing, pour lemon juice over it. It may sting, but it will stop the bleeding. To ease the sting, add water to the juice before pouring over the cut.

Sprinkle root of the *oshá* (lovage) plant on the cut.

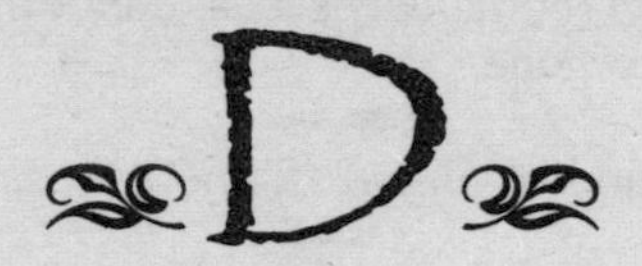

El que no llora no mama.

He who doesn't fuss isn't nursed.

DANDRUFF

To rid yourself of dandruff, grind an *aguacate* (avocado) pit and mix with *manteca* (lard). Rub the paste into your scalp and massage until your arms get tired. Cover your head with a cap or a towel and leave the paste on overnight. In the morning, wash your hair as usual.

DEPRESSION

Albahaca (basil) tea will soften your sorrow.

Damiana tea helps those who can't seem to shake the feeling of being depressed.

When suffering from feelings of desperation, drink *flor de tila* (linden flowers) tea.

DIABETES

Drink one of the following liquids when thirsty:
Sip on a tea made with the leaves of the *alcachofa* (artichoke) plant.

Drink a cold decoction of *aguacate* (avocado) peels thoughout the day, instead of water.

For diabetic infections, drink *maguey* (century plant) juice in water.

Sip damiana or *salvia* (sage) tea.

Drink *nopal* (prickly-pear cactus) water left out to catch the morning dew when you are thirsty.

Tronadora (trumpet flower) tea three times a day will work wonders.

In 1 liter of water, put 20 drops of your own urine. Drink in place of regular water.

DIAPER RASH

To relieve skin eruptions, pour a strained *malva* (mallow) infusion into the baby's bathwater.

Sprinkle pulverized dried *rosa de Castilla* (rose) petals on the baby's bottom.

Make an infusion of *ruda* (rue). Strain, then add to the baby's bathwater.

Pour a cup of *yerba mansa* (lizard tail) infusion into the baby's bathwater.

DIARRHEA (MOCTEZUMA'S REVENGE)

Drink a decoction of *aguacate* (avocado) bark until the diarrhea is relieved.

Drink a tea of 4 guava leaves seeped in 2 cups of water.

Simmer the bark and pods from the mesquite tree.

Eat the fruit called *tuna* from the *nopal* (prickly-pear cactus).

Sip a cup of warm, not hot, *estafiate* (wormwood) tea. This is safe enough for children (at ¼ dose).

DIGESTION

For better digestion, drink a decoction of *comino* (cumin) tea.

Take a *yerba buena* (mint) tincture, or just chew on the leaves and stems.

Drink a cold tea of *cuasia* (quassia).

Take a *romero* (rosemary) tincture in water or juice.

DISINFECTANT

Burn dried *alhucema* (lavender) petals in a room to clean the air of impurities. For generations, birthing rooms in homes have been disinfected in this manner.

Romero (rosemary) incense will disinfect the delivery room.

DIURETIC

See Water Retention

DRY SKIN

See Skin Care

DYSENTERY

Chew on *siempreviva* (stonecrop) leaves.

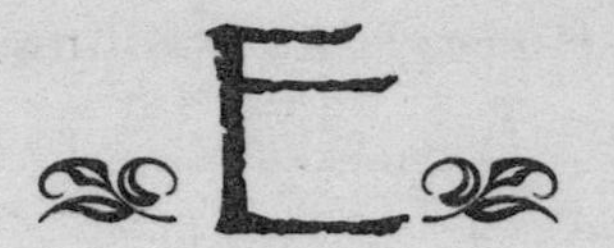

No hay mal que dure cien años
ni enfermo que lo aguante.

There is not a sickness that lasts one hundred years
nor a sick person who can endure it.

EARACHE

For pain or infection, apply two drops of hot *aceite de almendras* (almond oil) in the ailing ear, then tuck cotton in the ear.

Dip a couple of *albahaca* (basil) leaves in milk or oil, then insert into the ear.

Place a few drops of cayenne oil in the ear, then cover with cotton.

Heat 3 tablespoons dried *manzanilla* (chamomile) flowers in a ½ cup olive oil. Put a couple of drops in the ear, then cover with a cotton ball.

Put two or three *clavos* (cloves) in olive oil, then let steep for three or four days. Place a few drops in the ear, then cover with cotton. To speed the process, heat the *clavos* and oil in the microwave under the lowest setting until the oil is hot. Never substitute store-bought clove oil for this remedy. It will sting and be very painful.

Gently stick a raw, peeled *ajo* (garlic) clove in the ear. The thinner ones in the middle of the bulb work best.

Tuck a *punche* (Indian tobacco) leaf in the ear.

Heat a sliver of *cebolla* (onion) on a griddle and place it in the ear that hurts.

For this remedy you will need an assistant and a place safe from fire hazards. Pull hair and loose garments away from the affected ear. Wrap a good-sized piece of paper into a funnel and leave an opening at the bottom, just enough to fit into the ear. Tilt head sideways, place the funnel in the ear, and light the top of the funnel with a match. If you listen closely and remain motionless, you'll hear what seems like a huge rush of air escaping your ear. This will draw the cold air out of the ear, while balancing the fluids. When a sudden little puff of orange flame appears, remove the funnel and immediately place a cotton ball in the ear. Repeat on the other ear if both hurt. The ear pain will miraculously go away.

Place a *rosa de Castilla* (rose) petal in the infected ear.

A favorite remedy for earaches caused by head colds is to slowly heat 2 tablespoons olive oil. Add a few freshly bruised *ruda* (rue) leaves, then heat for a few minutes. Put a few drops of the warm oil into the ear, then cover with cotton.

If ears are ringing, sip on *ruda* (rue) tea.

Heat *siempreviva* (stonecrop) leaves and place in the ear.

Eczema

Apply fresh aloe vera gel to the skin.

Rinse skin with a *manzanilla* (chamomile) infusion instead of regular water.

Carefully rub *flor de San Juan* (evening primrose) oil onto the inflamed skin.

EMPACHO

Empacho *is the belief that food has lodged somewhere in the digestive tract, causing any number of intestinal problems, such as diarrhea, stomachache, loss of appetite, or vomiting. The patient is constantly thirsty, causing the belly to swell. It is more common with children, since they tend to swallow chewed gum and neglect to masticate their food properly.* Empacho *may also occur when hot and cold foods are improperly combined. Adults are also susceptible.*

Firmly rub an egg on the child's stomach. Where it breaks is where the knot is. Massage the knot with olive oil.

Simmer mesquite bark for 10 minutes, then drink.

Drink *yerba buena* (mint) tea.

Put 10 drops of a *romero* (rosemary) tincture in hot water, then drink.

If a child is suffering from *empacho*, have the child sip a cup of warm, not hot, *estafiate* (wormwood) tea.

Rub fresh chicken droppings on the calves, until the knots are gone.

ENERGY

Soak a handful of *aguja de piñon* (pine needles) overnight, strain, then add the liquid to your bath. This gives you the stamina you need to get through your day.

ESPANTO

The extreme of susto, espanto *happens while the body is abruptly forced into consciousness from a deep sleep. The soul may be drifting about, and not have time to get back to its host.* Espanto *may also result from falling out of bed or from a loud sound.*

Have the patient lie on a clean white sheet, then cover the patient up to the chin with another white sheet. The patient's arms should be extended, as if on the cross. Sweep the patient with a broom made of *romero* (rosemary), *marrubio* (horehound), and red bush branches. Recite the Apostles' Creed three times while sweeping the patient.

Simmer 1 teaspoon dried or 2 teaspoons fresh *cabellos de elote* (corn silk) in 2 cups of water until the water turns dark brown, then sip the entire two cups.

Drink a tea made with *epazote* (wormseed).

EYE INFLAMMATION

Place a *manzanilla* (chamomile) compress over the eyes.

Make a potato poultice by slicing or grating a potato. Mix in a teaspoon of warm water and apply over puffy eyelids.

EYE IRRITATION

According to folklore, rubbing breast milk on the eyes can ease irritation.

An eyewash of *rosa de Castilla* (rose) petals, water, and a pinch of salt will soothe eyes burned in the sweltering heat.

When eyes become irritated from the sun or dust, rinse eyes with urine, then water.

Rinse sore eyes with a cool *borraja* (borage) infusion.

Simmer mesquite pods and a pinch of salt in 2 cups water for 10 minutes. Once it is at room temperature, strain the liquid and use as an eye wash.

Boil 1 cup water and add ¼ teaspoon salt. This is a good saline solution. Let cool, then use. Make fresh daily.

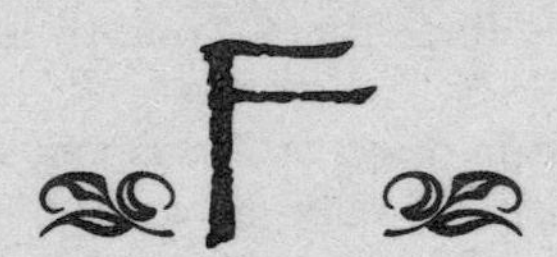

Cada uno sabe dónde le aprieta el zapato.

Each one knows where the shoe pinches him.

Feet

Soak sore, tired feet in *salvado* (bran) and hot water.

Soak feet in freshly grated *ajengibre* (ginger) and hot water.

Fertility

Frío en la matriz, *or cold uterus, occurs when the new mother does not get enough rest. She may experience irregular periods and a disinterest in sex.*

For *frío en la matriz*, sip on damiana tea every morning, starting with the last day of your period. Continue to drink for two weeks.

Drink *salvia* (sage) tea every morning for two weeks.

Fever

Teas are not only therapeutic but nurturing when you are running a fever. Mix the following herbs to create your own blend:

Ajengibre (ginger root) tea

Azafrán (safflower) tea

Canela (cinnamon bark) tea

Eucalipto (eucalyptus) tea

Flor saúco (elder flowers) tea

Fresh _fresno_ (ash) leaves tea

Gordolobo (mullein) leaves tea

Hot lemonade with honey

Té de limón (lemongrass tea)

Rub a tincture of fresh *fresno* (ash) leaves and tequila all over the patient, then bundle in warm blankets. Place the leaves on the forehead of the patient, and remove only after they have dried. Allow the patient to get plenty of rest.

Drink a decoction made with *álamo* (aspen) bark and leaves.

To help reduce fever, make an enema by mixing 1 teaspoon *carbonato* (baking soda) with 1 pint warm water.

For fevers accompanied by bronchial infection, drink a lukewarm *borraja* (borage) tea.

For a fever accompanied by a headache, rub the body with an *alcanfor* (camphor) and mescal (peyote) tincture, then bundle up in blankets. Once the patient is tucked into bed, place an *alcanfor* poultice on the forehead. Sleep will no doubt follow.

Make an infusion of *oshá* (lovage) plant. Strain and add to your bathwater.

Kill a young black hen, then cut it into several pieces. Apply the pieces to the chest while they are still warm.

Spread a *plantilla* (foot poultice) of tequila and mustard seeds to the soles of the feet, then cover with loose cotton socks or gauze.

Soak *encino* (oak) leaves and branches for a full day, then drink the liquid when thirsty.

Peel and thinly slice a potato. Soak the slices in vinegar and salt, then place on the forehead. Hold in place with a cloth, folded to about two inches wide, that will comfortably fit around the head. Somehow, the potatoes absorb the fever and will make you feel a lot better within an hour or two. Take the potato slices off when they became warm.

Drink an infusion of yellow *rosa de Castilla* (rose) petals at room temperature. Add sugar to taste. A weak tea is safe for children as well.

Wet the tips of your fingers with saliva and make the sign of the cross on the patient's forehead and the bottom of the feet. This will take the evil (fever) out of the patient. Somehow it always seems to work!

This remedy for fevers was used by my great grandmother. The process is simple, but you must keep in mind that if the fever is accompanied by a cold, it is best not to use it until the cold is gone. You will need a bucket full of extremely cold water that comes a little higher than the patient's knees, a towel, and blankets. To start off, the patient takes off his or her shoes and socks and places his or her feet inside the water for approximately two minutes. Immediately dry the feet and keep them warm in the towel for three minutes. This procedure is repeated three to five times, after which the patient is bundled in the blankets. The fever will have dropped and the patient should sleep for a good six to eight hours.

When you have a fever and suffer from a headache, drink a decoction of 1 part *jarita* (willow bark) and 5 parts water, three times a day. This will sweat the fever out and clear the head.

When you have a fever, make a tea with the leaves and flower tops of the *plumajillo* (yarrow) plant. Not only will this tangy drink get rid of the chills, but it will help sweat out the illness. Drink three times a day.

FINGERNAILS

See Nails

FLATULENCE

To prevent embarrassing flatulence, sip on the following teas:

Anís **(aniseed) tea**

Anís de estrella **(star anise) tea**

Alhucema **(lavender) tea**

Comino **(cumin) tea**

Drink a cup of *hinojo* (fennel) seeds simmered in milk.

Pulverize *nuez moscada* (nutmeg), simmer in water for about 10 minutes, then drink the liquid.

Chew on a slice of raw *cebolla* (onion).

Flu

Sip on *manzanilla* (chamomile), lemon, and honey tea.

Sip *eucalipto* (eucalyptus) tea and inhale the vapors.

When you are just coming down with the flu, take a *yerba del indio* (Indian root) tincture and go straight to bed.

Freckles

Rub a *flor de San Juan* (evening primrose) petal on the freckles, and watch them fade.

Frostbite

Soak frostbitten fingers or toes in *marrubio* (horehound) leaves and hot water, until water is lukewarm.

Fumigation

Burn dried *alhucema* (lavender) petals in your home to clean the air of impurities. For generations, maternity rooms in homes have been fumigated in this manner.

Fumigate your home by simmering *tomillo* (thyme) in a big pot.

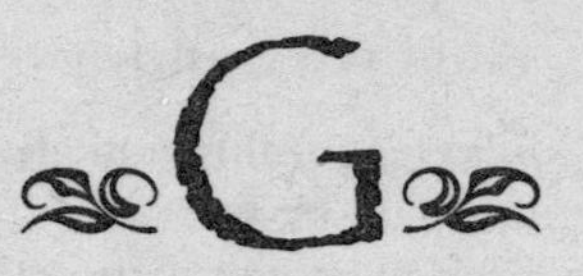

Es mejor prevenir que lamentar.

It is better to prevent than to lament.

Gallstones

Put a handful of bruised *gordolobo* (mullein) leaves in a pint of water, then let stand for three days. Drink 3 cups a day.

Gas

A teaspoon of *carbonato* (baking soda) in a glass of water will relieve the pain of gas.

Drink *albahaca* (basil) leaf tea.

Drink a cup of hot water (as hot as you can stand it) with the juice from a half of a lemon.

Gums

When gums are sore, grind an *aguacate* (avocado) pit, then place a pinch of its meat on the gum, just as if it were tobacco.

To rid gums of pain and swelling, boil *cilantro* (coriander) seeds, strain, and rinse the mouth with this decoction.

To stop gums from bleeding, chew on fresh *perejil* (parsley).

Gargle with a *salvia* (sage) infusion at room temperature.

To maintain healthy gums and teeth, chew on the root of the *yerba mansa* (lizard tail) plant.

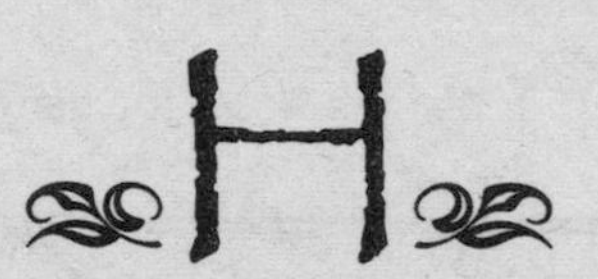

Mientras que la hierba crece el caballo no muere.

As long as grass grows the horse won't die.

Hair

To speed hair growth, mash the fruit of an *aguacate* (avocado), then apply the paste to your scalp. Leave on overnight, then wash as usual.

After washing your hair, rinse with the essence of *manzanilla* (chamomile) flowers. This will keep hair shiny and fragrant.

A *culantrillo* (maidenhair fern) hair rinse will help hair maintain its shine. Just rinse clean hair with a strained infusion.

Hangover

To prevent, or at least minimize, a hangover, drink *oshá* (lovage) tea before you drink the hard stuff.

When you have drunk too much or mixed liquors that didn't get along, drink a cup of tea made with alfalfa seeds.

Combine *clavos* (cloves), *nuez moscada* (nutmeg), *canela* (cinnamon), and *yerba buena* (mint) in a decoction and sip.

Atole (corn gruel) is always good for hangovers.

Drink a *canela* (cinnamon bark) and *ajengibre* (ginger) decoction.

To clear out a hangover, make a decoction from fresh *ajengibre* (ginger) root. Drink it straight: no cream, no sugar.

Hung over? Make a tea with orange and lemon blossoms and leaves.

Yerba maté tea will get you through work when you are really hung over.

Drink a tea made from the flowers of the *uña de gato* (catclaw) shrub.

Menudo is always good for *el crudo* (hangover).

Harelip

A woman can avoid giving birth to a child with a harelip by wearing a safety pin on her underwear throughout her pregnancy.

Hay Fever

Drink *cañutillo* (Mormon tea) slowly, so that you inhale the vapors.

To relieve itchy eyes and sneezing, drink *yerba santa* (mountain balm) tea.

HEADACHE

It is the custom in Mexico to apply leaves of the following plants directly onto the temples when suffering from a headache. They are kept in place with saliva or the syrupy liquid that some of the plants secrete. The leaves may also be crushed and mixed with salt and oil, then rubbed into the temples.

Llantén **(plantain)**

Perejil **(parsley)**

Punche **(Indian tobacco)**

Ruda **(rue)**

Siempreviva **(stonecrop)**

Toloache **(jimson weed)**

Uña de gato **(catclaw)**

Yerba buena **(mint)**

Lie down and apply an *alcanfor* (camphor) and *mescal* (peyote) poultice on the forehead.

Heat dried *hediondilla* (chaparral) leaves and lard. Strain into a jar with a lid. Once the mixture is at room temperature, rub it into the temples.

For headaches caused by hunger, drink a cup of hot chocolate made with water instead of milk.

Drink a strong cup of black coffee.

When a headache is caused by sinus infection, take a steam inhalation of laurel leaves.

Calabaza (pumpkin) pulp makes a good poultice for headaches.

Rub a *ruda* (rue) tincture onto your temples.

For reading headaches, place an *alfafón* (sweet clover) poultice over the eyes. Rest until the headache is gone.

Pour hot water over *tomillo* (thyme). Strain and drink the liquid when it is cold.

When you have a fever and suffer from a headache, drink a decoction of 1 part *jarita* (willow bark) and 5 parts water, three times a day. This will sweat the fever out and clear the head.

Thinly slice a potato, dip in vinegar and apply to forehead. The potatoes can be kept in place with a towel. Lie down in a dark, quiet room until headache is gone.

Make an infusion of *estafiate* (wormwood) leaves, strain, then add to a tub of hot water. Soak in the tub until the headache is gone.

Heart Tonics

To keep your heart beating strong and steady, drink *flor saúco* (elder flowers) tea.

Heartburn

When too much good food gives you heartburn, drink a cup of *angélica* tea as needed.

HEATSTROKE

Have the patient lie down in the shade and drink salted water. Apply a compress dipped in an infusion of cool *saúco* (elder) flowers and leaves.

HEMORRHOIDS

Peel off the outer layer of the aloe vera leaf and apply to the hemorrhoid.

Take a sitz bath in lukewarm water and aloe vera extract.

Heat tender *saúco* (elder) leaves in olive oil, then apply to the hemorrhoid.

Bruise a *toloache* (jimson weed) leaf, coat it with lard, and place it on the hemorrhoid.

Apply a *gordolobo* (mullein) poultice to the affected area.

Take a sitz bath in an infusion of *yerba mansa* (lizard tail). Then apply a poultice of *yerba mansa* leaves on the hemorrhoid.

HICCUPS

When the baby has hiccups, you can relieve them by using saliva to stick a piece of wound-up red thread on the baby's forehead. Within a few minutes the hiccups will be gone.

Pour sugar on half a lemon or lime and squeeze into the mouth.

Hives

Boil 1 tablespoon of *zarzaparrilla* (sarsaparilla) root in 1 cup of water, strain, and drink.

Hot Flashes

See Menopause

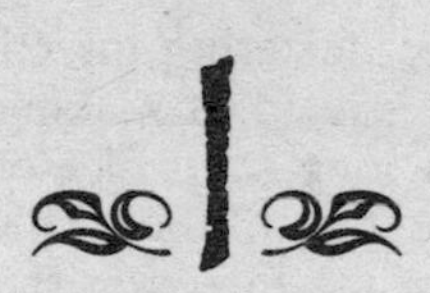

No hay mal que por bien no venga.

There is no ill that good can't come from.

Impotence

Drink damiana tea every day for two weeks, and again before becoming intimate.

Drink ½ cup of *raíz del Macho* (muira puama) tea first thing in the morning until desired results are obtained. This should not take too long.

Indigestion

As soon as you are done with a spicy or heavy meal, chew on *anís* (aniseed). This will help you to digest your food and keep you from feeling bloated.

Drink *alhucema* (lavender) and honey tea.

Drink an *ajengibre* (ginger) decoction to ease an upset stomach.

Eat a slice of papaya after a heavy meal to detour indigestion.

Infections (external)

Take care of a large, festering infection by boiling some *masa* (cornmeal). Instead of making a tamale, spread it in the center of a long strip of cloth and wrap it over the infection while it is still hot. The next day, the swelling and rawness of the infection should be gone.

Infertility

Drink *salvia* (sage) or damiana tea every morning for 2 weeks.

Insect Bites

Keep an aloe vera tincture in the cupboard and apply to mosquito bites or anything that itches.

When a red ant bites you, spread some *barro* (mud) on the bite. The cool mud stops the itching.

Immediately after being bitten, cut a clove of raw *ajo* (garlic) in half, then dip it in salt. Apply directly to the bite. The garlic will not only draw the venom out, but it will also keep the swelling down.

To get rid of the itch quick, take a fresh jalapeño and rub it on a mosquito bite.

Pour salt on a slice of lime or lemon, then heat on a griddle. Place the hot slice (salt side down) on the affected area. This will take the itch out and reduce swelling.

Bruise a *llantén* (plantain) leaf, then apply to the insect bite.

Make a potato poultice by slicing or grating a potato. Mix in a teaspoon of cold water and apply to the bite.

Dip the insect bite in hot salted water.

Rub tequila and salt on the insect bite.

Insect Repellent

Apply a tincture of raw *ajo* (garlic) liberally to exposed skin.

Simmer laurel leaves in your home to keep the insects out.

Simmer the pulp and seeds from the *calabazilla* (wild gourd) plant, strain, then pour into a spray bottle.

Simmer *plumajillo* (yarrow) in water, then strain. Once it has cooled, spray on skin.

Insomnia

Having trouble falling asleep? A tincture of herbs under the tongue, or a nice hot cup of one of the following teas, will put you out for the night. Best of all, your head will not have that vacant feeling the next morning:

***Anís de estrella* (star anise) tea**
***Borraja* (borage) tea**
***Flor de tila* (linden flowers) tea**
***Manzanilla* (chamomile) tea**
***Pasionaria* (passionflower) tea**
***Salvia* (sage) tea**
***Valeriana* (valerian) root tea**

To ensure a good night's sleep, soak in a tub of *flor de tila* (linden flowers).

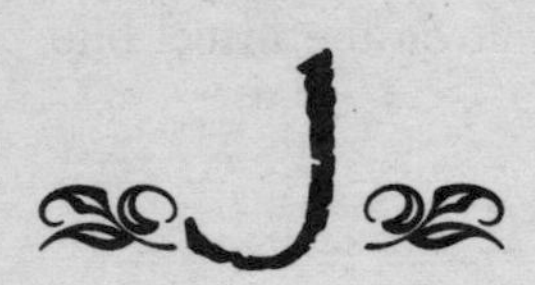

Olvidar la injuria es el mejor venganza.

Forgetting the injury is the best revenge.

JELLYFISH STINGS

Place a cold papaya poultice on the jellyfish sting.

JOINTS

To ease the pain of swollen joints, soak *aguja de piñon* (pine needles) overnight, strain, then add the liquid to your bath.

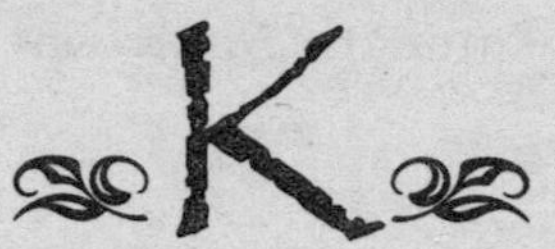

El que paga el médico es el que cura.

He who pays the physician does the cure.

Kidney Disorders

Drink 3 cups of alfalfa tea every day for two weeks. This will flush out your system and strengthen your kidneys.

To flush out your kidneys, make a tea with *manzanilla* (chamomile) and *cabellos de elote fresco* (fresh corn silk). Drink every morning for one week.

Sip on a decoction of *hediondilla* (chaparral). If the tea is unpalatable, which I'm sure it will be, take a tincture of 15 drops in its place.

Simmer a whole *flor de San Juan* (evening primrose flower) with 1 cup water for 5-10 minutes and drink.

It is believed that *grano de lino* (flaxseed) tea will help many kidney complaints.

Drink a decoction of *cola de caballo* (horsetail) roots. Make enough to last the day, keep it in the refrigerator, and drink it when you are thirsty. This will rid the body of too much liquid and clear the kidneys.

Kidney Stones

To rid the body of impurities, drink a warm decoction of *chicória* (dandelion) root tea. This will break down kidney stones.

To dissolve kidney stones, prepare *cañutillo* (Mormon tea). Drink 1 cup on an empty stomach. Repeat for twelve days.

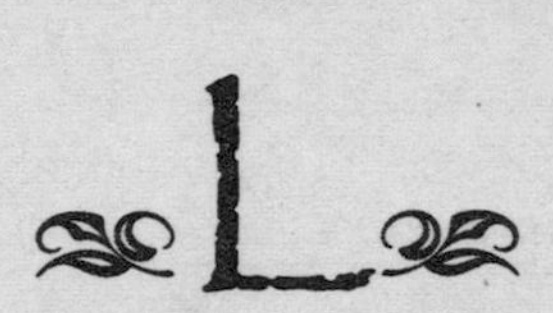

Una madre es para cien hijos,
pero cien hijos no son para una madre.

One mother can take care of one hundred sons;
one hundred sons can not take care of one mother.

Labor

To help induce labor, drink a decoction of *álamo* (aspen) bark and leaves. Be sure that the house is in order and that the others are taken care of before the first sip.

Drink *yerba buena* (mint) tea before delivery to hasten birth.

Once labor has been induced, have the mother-to-be drink *albahaca* (basil) tea between contractions. This will cut her pain.

When childbearing becomes painful and strenuous, a *comino* (cumin) decoction should be sipped between labor pains. This will stimulate the uterus.

To speed up childbirth, cook a chopped *cebolla* (onion) in lard, then remove from heat. Add dried *manzanilla* (chamomile) flowers and mix thoroughly. While it is still warm, rub it over the body. After giving birth, the new mother should drink *manzanilla* tea, with a pinch of *carbonato* (baking soda). This will flush out her womb.

LACTATION

To stimulate lactation, the new mother should sip a tea of *anís* (aniseed) or a decoction of *hinojo* (fennel) seeds.

When a woman gives birth, her first milk may be rejected by the baby. If this happens, the mother should drink *alhucema* (lavender) tea. Before attempting to nurse the infant again, dip the nipple in the tea, then nurse.

Sip *yerba buena* (mint) tea.

Drink 1 cup *epazote* (wormseed) tea every day until lactation is stimulated.

LAUNDRY SOAP

Simmer the pulp and seeds from the *calabazilla* (wild gourd) plant, strain, then bottle.

LEECHES

A surefire way to force a leech to release its grip is to burn it off with a lit cigarette.

LICE

Wash hair in vinegar, then comb out.

Liver Disorders

Grind and simmer roots of *chicória* (dandelion), then drink the liquid warm to stimulate the liver and flush the bowels.

Boil young lime leaves, lime rind, sugar, and water. Strain and drink. The liquid cleans out the impurities in the liver.

Drink *tronadora* (trumpet flower) tea.

Liver Spots

Twice a day, apply fresh aloe vera gel to those brown spots that you get on the back of your hand.

Luck

If you run out of salt, you run out of good luck, so always check to see if you are low before going to the grocery store.

Lung Conditions

Kill a young black hen, then cut it into several pieces. Apply the pieces to the chest while they are still warm.

Place one raw *cebolla morada* (purple onion), quartered, and 5 tablespoons honey into the blender. Blend on low speed for 3 seconds. Leave the mixture in a bowl, loosely covered, by an open window (or outside to catch the morning dew) overnight. Take 2 spoonfuls of the liquid every two hours until better.

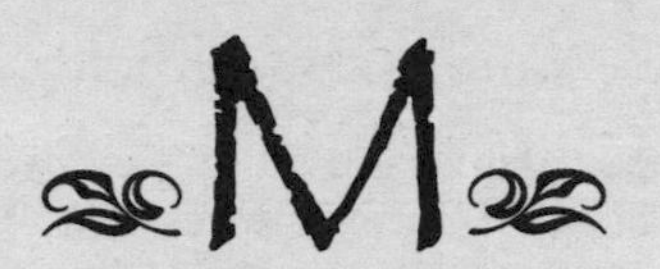

El que mucho mal
padece con poco bien se conforma.

He who suffers many evils
is comforted with just a little good.

Mal de Ojo (The Evil Eye)

Contrary to its name, the evil eye is caused by excessive admiration. The evil eye is most common among infants, since they are young and are believed to be unable to take such strong adoration. If a stranger admires a baby, the stranger must touch the infant in order to invoke God's protection from the evil eye. If not touched, the baby will experience a high fever, a lack of appetite or sleep, and vomiting. Mal de ojo *can be transferred by anyone.*

To avert *mal de ojo,* drink *anís* (aniseed) tea.

A good way to protect yourself and your children from *mal de ojo* is to carry an amulet of *ojo de venado* (horse chestnut/buckeye) when out in public. The *ojo de venado* is not the eye of a deer but a seed.

Though the cures for the evil eye vary, the most common cure is to rub an egg (at room temperature) all over the body of the child while saying three Our Fathers or the Apostles' Creed in Spanish or English. You can have the child either lie down or stand up during the process. When finished, get a glass filled halfway with water (clear glass with no designs on it), and slowly crack the egg in it. Place the egg under the bed, directly beneath the child's head. Have the child sleep over the egg for one night. This will draw the evil out. In the morning, examine the egg. If the egg looks cooked or the yolk has the orange image of an eye, the diagnosis is positive.

Measles

To precipitate the outgrowth of measles, apply an *alcanfor* (camphor), lard, and *carbonato* (baking soda) paste to the skin.

There is no way around the measles once you get them. To bolster the eruptions, drink a cold infusion of *azafrán* (safflower) or sip on *flor saúco* (elder flowers) tea.

Menopause

An *anís* (aniseed) bath will cool hot flashes. Just add a strained infusion to your bathwater.

Menstrual Cramps

Sip a tea of *aguacate* (avocado) leaves, hot or cold, to relieve menstrual cramping.

Sip *albahaca* (basil) tea not only to bring relief from menstrual cramps, but also to help keep your period on schedule.

Drink *epazote* (wormseed) tea to bring about your period and ease cramping as well.

Drink *yerba mansa* (lizard tail) tea to relieve cramps.

Menstrual Flow (heavy)

If your menstrual flow is heavy, sip on a *consuelda* (comfrey) decoction.

Make *plumajillo* (yarrow) tea when menstrual flow is heavy and cramps are strong. Drink three times a day.

A *sabino* (juniper) needles sitz bath works wonders to lighten a heavy flow. Just make a decoction with the needles, and strain into a shallow basin of water.

Menstrual Stimulant

A good way to bring about your period without provoking cramps is to drink a *culantrillo* (maidenhair fern) root decoction.

Drink *romero* (rosemary) tea.

When you feel achy and heavy with cramps, but your period won't start, sip ½ cup *ruda* (rue) tea. This will also keep your period regular.

Drink *epazote* (wormseed) tea to bring on your period and to ease cramping.

Migraine

Inhale the fragrant *hinojo* (fennel) vapors to soothe a migraine, or place a poultice of the seeds on your eyes, and try to relax.

Miscarriage

Alhucemo (lavender) and *manzanilla* (chamomile) tea is a good way to ease the sorrow of a miscarriage.

Drink tea made with *manzanilla* in which a gold ring has been boiled.

Morning Sickness

To curb morning sickness, try the following teas:

Ajengibre (ginger) tea

Canela (cinnamon bark) tea

Yerba buena (mint) tea

Mosquito Bites

See Insect Bites

Moth Repellent

Alfafón (sweet clover) in drawers and trunks will keep the moths away.

Mouthwash

Instead of buying mouthwash, try simmered and strained *borraja* (borage) leaves and seeds.

Mumps

Apply sliced potatoes smeared with lard under the ears, then wrap into place with gauze.

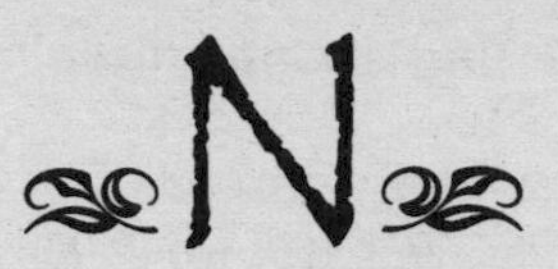

Un médico crea trabajo para otro médico.

One doctor makes work for another doctor.

Nails

To strengthen nails, rub a clove of raw *ajo* (garlic) on the fingernails every day.

To remedy weak nails, rub in a dab of olive oil on the surface of the clean, unpolished nails. Repeat daily.

Nausea

Whenever you feel like you're going to throw up, put a pinch of *carbonato* (baking soda) on your tongue. Drink ½ cup water. You should feel better in less than 10 seconds.

Sip *canela* (cinnamon bark) and honey tea.

Drink a decoction of *clavos* (cloves). A few drops of *aceite de clavos* (clove oil) on the tongue should help as well.

Drink a cup of black coffee that has been stirred with a *canela* (cinnamon) stick instead of a spoon.

For any kind of nausea, including morning sickness, drink *ajengibre* (ginger) tea.

Chew on fresh *yerba buena* (mint).

Neck Stiffness

Place a poultice of *yerba santa* (mountain balm) and lard on the neck.

Nerves

To soothe the nerves, drink one of the following teas:

Apio (celery) seed tea

Lemon blossom tea

Salvia (sage) tea

Valeriana (valerian) root tea

Brew a *cilantro* (coriander) seed tea, then drink the decoction as needed. This is safe for children.

Drink a tea made from the blossoms and the rind of the orange to relax the nerves.

Drink a tea made from the flowers of the *uña de gato* (catclaw) shrub.

Drink a weak tea of *girasol* (sunflower) to calm the nerves. It is very important not to use much of the plant, because it is very potent and can create unpleasant stomach disturbances.

Nightmares

A glass of water underneath your children's beds will protect them from bad dreams.

Nosebleeds

Make a poultice out of fresh *lama del agua* (algae). Tilt head back and place poultice behind the neck. Remove the poultice when the bleeding stops. You'll notice that the algae has dried and turned yellow.

Fresh *perejil* (parsley) stuck up the nose will stop bleeding.

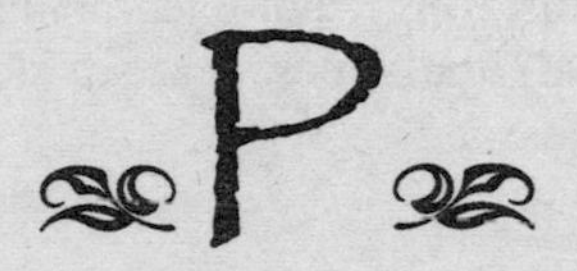

Salud y alegría belleza crian.

Health and happiness create beauty.

PIMPLES

Simmer *malva* (mallow), *salvado* (bran), and water in a saucepan. Strain the mixture and use as a rinse three times a day. Drape the face with a hot towel that has been soaked in a decoction of *malva* (mallow) and *salvado* (bran).

Mash *hediondilla* (chaparral) leaves, then apply to pimples.

Wash face, then splash with a *consuelda* (comfrey) rinse. Next, dab a cotton ball soaked in a tincture of *consuelda* (comfrey) on the pimples.

Wash face then rinse with a tincture of *flor saúco* (elder flowers).

Pinkeye (Conjunctivitis)

Wash the child's eye out with breast milk.

Pneumonia

When you are suffering from pneumonia, make *anís* (aniseed) tea. Inhale the vapors and sip slowly.

Poison Ivy

To get rid of the itch quick, place a bruised *llantén* (plantain) leaf directly on the irritated area of skin.

Postpartum Care

After she gives birth, allow the new mother a few sips of *epazote* (wormseed) tea. This will help alleviate the pains that follow childbirth.

The new mother should also drink *canela* (cinnamon bark) tea. This will reduce the contractions that follow delivery.

Pregnancy

See Labor, Morning Sickness, and Postpartum Care.

Psoriasis

Make an ointment with *consuelda* (comfrey) and lard, then apply to the skin.

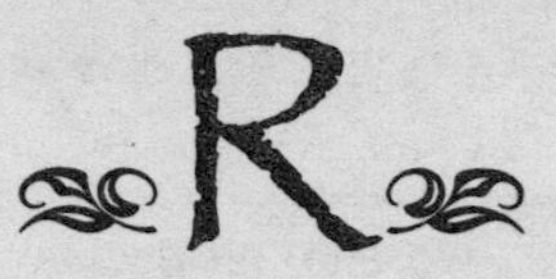

Hay veces que nada el pato, y hay otras que ni agua bebe.

There are times when the duck swims in the water, and others when he won't even drink it.

Rattlesnake Bite

A good rattlesnake repellent is the root of the *oshá* (lovage) plant. If you find yourself in the desert, keep the root in hand. At night, scatter the pulverized root around your campsite.

If you are bitten, rinse the bite with water or urine; fasten a tourniquet between the bite and the heart and loosen every 20 minutes for 20 seconds. Cut two cross-incisions (avoid veins and arteries) ½ inch long and ¼ inch deep at each fang puncture, suck the venom out, and spit. Apply a *toloache* (jimson weed) poultice on the bite and get to the hospital immediately.

Respiratory Problems

Inhale *hediondilla* (chaparral) steam.

Make a tea and a poultice from the leaves and flowers of the *gordolobo* (mullein) plant and place it on the chest. This will relax the chest, allowing comfortable breathing.

Apply a *cebolla* (onion) and hot vinegar compress or poultice on the chest.

Rheumatism

Rub an *aguacate* (avocado) pit tincture on the aches.

Rub *aceite de linas* (linseed oil) on the skin, then cover with *punche* (Indian tobacco) leaves. Wrap with gauze to keep in place.

Massage a tincture of tequila and green marijuana on the affected area, then cover with a flannel cloth.

Make a tincture with alcohol and minced dried peyote. Place the liquid in a dark cupboard for a week. Rub the solution onto the affected area.

Boil a dried *girasol* (sunflower) in a pot of water, strain, then add to a warm bath. Soak until the pain is eased. After your bath, rub a tincture of *girasol* (sunflower) where needed.

Shave a dog, then sleep with the animal until you feel better.

Ringworm

As soon as you wake up in the morning, before you speak a word, rub saliva on the affected skin.

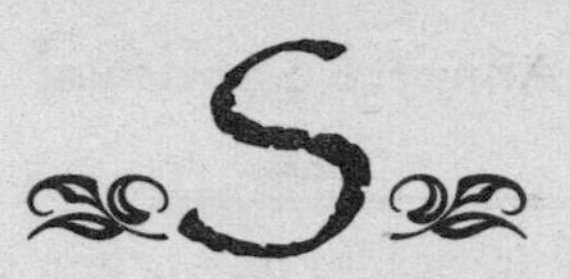

El que con leche se quema
hasta al jocoque le sopla.

He who is burned by milk
is even afraid of cottage cheese.

Scalds

Cover the area with a minced raw *cebolla* (onion), then wrap with a clean cloth. Not only will it alleviate the pain, but it will prevent the burn from blistering.

Grind fresh *siempreviva* (stonecrop) leaves in a mortar and pestle, then apply on the scalded area. Wrap with gauze.

Scars

Squeeze half a lemon into a mother-of-pearl shell; you'll notice that the juice thickens to a paste. Dab the paste on the scar twice a day. Add a bit of patience, as scars fade slowly.

Make a tincture with *aguja de piñon* (pine needles) and alcohol and let stand until the liquid turns green (a week or two). Apply to the scar daily until the scar cannot be found.

Scorpion Stings

If you are bitten by a scorpion, kill the little nuisance, then apply his guts onto the sting until you reach a doctor.

Scrapes

Before applying the bandage, place a spiderweb on the clean scrape.

Dab a *yerba mansa* (lizard tail) root tincture on the scrape. This will keep it from getting infected.

Seasickness

As soon as the boat is launched, start sucking on cinnamon- or ginger-flavored hard candy.

Shampoo

For really clean hair, simmer *calabazilla* (wild gourd) fruit and pulp, then strain into empty shampoo bottles. Use every day.

Amole (yucca) extract makes a good shampoo. Simmer equal parts chopped *amole* and cold water until liquid becomes thick. Strain into an airtight container.

Sinus Infection

Steam the leaves and bark of the *álamo* (aspen) tree in water, then breathe the vapors in through your nose.

Inhale the steam of an *ajengibre* (ginger) decoction as you sip it.

Inhale the vapors of lemon leaves in water, then sip slowly.

Steam *yerba mansa* (lizard tail) root in an enclosed room.

Sip on a tea made with *yerba santa* (mountain balm) leaves throughout the day. This should clear the sinuses.

Skin Cancer

Heat dried *hediondilla* (chaparral) leaves and lard. Strain into a jar and cover. Once the mixture has cooled to room temperature, rub it onto the affected area as needed.

Boil *encino* (oak) bark for 10 minutes. Once it has cooled, wash the affected area with this water.

Skin Care

For a face that glows, mash the fruit of an *aguacate* (avocado), then apply the paste to your skin. Leave it on for 15 minutes, then rinse with warm water. Do this once a week, or more often if you have the time. You'll notice a difference right away.

Splash an infusion of *rosa de Castilla* (rose) petals liberally on your skin to bring out its glow.

To subdue wrinkles, make a decoction from bruised *romero* (rosemary) leaves and flowers. Add to your bathwater or use as a facial rinse. This is a good facial astringent.

Soap

Liquid soap is really easy to make. All you need is 1 part fresh *amole* (yucca) root to 2 parts water simmered until water thickens.

Sore Muscles

See Aches

Sore Throat

When your throat is so swollen that you are having difficulty swallowing your own saliva, gargle with a strong infusion of hot *albahaca* (basil), salt, and water.

Make a poultice from *flor de San Juan* (evening primrose) flowers and hot oil. Wrap over throat.

Mix a shot of tequila, 1 or 2 tablespoons of honey, and the juice from a lemon. Swallow slowly; try to let the liquid coat your throat as it goes down.

Gargle with a strong decoction of *raíz del Macho* (muira puama) bark.

Boil *cañaigre* roots, strain, and gargle with the liquid when it has cooled to room temperature.

Pulverize the dried red petals of a *rosa de Castilla* (rose), and mix with oil. Coat the throat with the mixture. For a quick fix, pluck a few fresh petals and place on the tongue.

Gargle with hot salt water.

Take 1 tablespoon honey with minced *tomillo* (thyme) every morning and evening until symptoms are gone.

Sip on *yerba santa* (mountain balm) tea with honey and lemon.

Speed

Egg whites on the back of the knees will ensure that a baby will run fast when he or she gets older.

Spider Bites

First, draw the poison out; then crush an *aguacate* (avocado) pit and add lard and baking soda. Apply to the spider bite.

Chew on a *gordolobo* (mullein) leaf, then place it on the spider bite.

Splinters

To remove a splinter, heat *trementina de piñon* (pine pitch) and spread it over the splinter. Peel it off when it cools and hardens.

Split Ends

Rub *aguacate* (avocado) oil onto the tips of the hair shafts to reduce split ends.

Sprains

Massage a sprain with a tincture or salve of dried arnica flowers and rhizomes. This will reduce the pain and bring down any swelling.

Combine chopped *toloache* (jimson weed) and heated lard. Apply the poultice to the sprain. Wrap with gauze.

Stiff Neck

See Neck Stiffness

Stomachache

Ease stomach pains with the following herbs:

Ajengibre **(ginger) decoction**
Alfalfa seed tea
Alhucema **(lavender) tea**
Angélica tea
Apio **(celery) seeds tea**
Canela **(cinnamon) tea**
Cañutillo **(Mormon tea) twigs tea**
Cascara sagrada **root tea**
Epazote **(Mexican) tea**
Malva **(mallow) root tea**
Manzanilla **(chamomile) tea**
Oshá **(lovage) tea**
Plumajillo **(yarrow) tea**
Siempreviva **(stonecrop) tea**
Té de limón **(lemongrass tea)**
Uña de gato **(catclaw) tea**
Valeriana **(valerian) root tea**
Yerba buena **(mint) tea**

Atole (corn gruel) is always good for an upset stomach.

Drink a cold infusion of *marrubio* (horehound) leaves and honey until you feel better.

Place a poultice of *yerba del indio* (Indian root) on the stomach.

When you feel sick *de la pansa* (to your stomach) with a little bit of fever, pluck a handful of *rosa de Castilla* (rose) petals. Make into a tea and add honey. This will help you to relax. When you wake up you'll feel a lot better.

Pulverize *nuez moscada* (nutmeg), simmer in water for about 10 minutes, strain, then drink.

Take a *yerba mansa* (lizard tail) tincture.

Place 15 drops of an *estafiate* (wormwood) tincture under the tongue.

Place a *yerba mansa* (lizard tail) poultice on the tummy.

Stress

When you experience feelings of tension and can't relax, drink a nice hot cup of *anís* (aniseed) tea with honey or *té de limón* (lemon grass tea).

Sty

Poke a needle halfway into the seed of a lemon, then heat. Apply the hot seed directly on the outside of the sty.

Sunburn

Mash a bowl of cooked and cooled *frijoles* (beans). Smear the paste onto the sunburn.

Make a potato poultice by slicing or grating a potato. Mix in a teaspoon of cold water and apply to the sunburn.

To soothe a sunburn and keep it from peeling, slice off the outer layer of a *nopal* (prickly-pear cactus) and apply the plant ooze onto the sunburn.

To cool a sunburn, use a vinegar compress.

SUSTO

The syndrome known as susto, *or fright, is the loss of the spirit or soul due to a sudden shock.* Susto *may occur after a sudden fright, such as witnessing an accident or a sudden fall. This shock loosens the* alma, *or soul, from the body. Though nearby, the* alma *needs to be lured back into its person by means of herbs and rituals. The longer this illness goes untreated, the more serious the condition becomes. The symptoms include anorexia, lethargy, and depression. This disease appears to be native to the Americas, with children and pregnant women being more susceptible to its influences.*

Make an *anís* (aniseed) tincture. Take 20 drops three times a day until you are better.

Sip *albahaca* (basil) tea or *canela* (cinnamon bark) and honey tea.

Place *marrubio* (horehound) under your pillow, between the mattresses, or under the bed to keep *susto* away and permit a safe night's sleep.

This process has to be done on Wednesday, Thursday, and Friday, after 7:00 P.M. Once the process has begun, the patient cannot go outside until Saturday. You'll need three lemons at room temperature (a different lemon is used for each day) and a crucifix.

First, have the patient take a spoonful of sugar followed by a glass of water. The patient must then lie down in bed and be covered with a white blanket. Hold one of the lemons and the crucifix in one hand and make small cross patterns all over the body—from head to toes. Chant "Come (say patient's name), don't go, Virgin Mother help her" three times, and repeat three more times. On Friday night, place the three lemons and the crucifix under the pillow of the patient. Then, on Saturday morning before daybreak, throw the lemons in the street, at an intersection.

Drink *romero* (rosemary) tea.

Perform a *barrida* (sweeping). Have the patient explain the cause of the *susto*, then lie on a clean white sheet. Cover the patient up to the chin with another white sheet. The patient's arms should be extended, as if on the cross. Sweep the patient with a broom made of *romero* (rosemary) or *marrubio* (horehound) branches. Recite the Apostles' Creed three times while sweeping the patient. Do this every third day until the patient is better. For best results, start the barrida on a Wednesday or a Friday.

When you have had to endure a serious trauma, and are left with a lingering feeling of anguish and despair, bathe in an infusion of *flor de tila* (linden) tea. This will calm the memories.

SWELLING

Combine chopped *toloache* (jimson weed) and heated lard. Apply the poultice to the swelling. Wrap with gauze.

Crush a handful of green *llantén* (plantain) leaves and mix with ½ cup olive oil. Apply the poultice on the affected area, then wrap with gauze or clean rags.

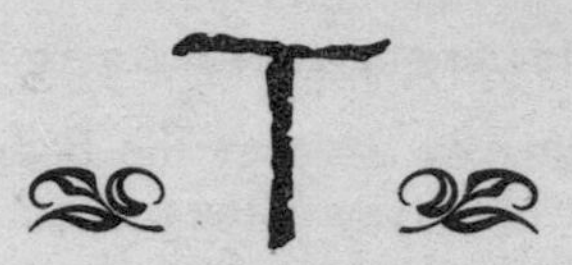

El que paga lo que debe,
sana del mal que padece.

He who pays his debts
recovers from the illness that he suffers.

Tapeworms

An old remedy for ridding the body of tapeworms is to make a decoction from a handful of *pepitas* (pumpkin seeds). Drink the decoction at room temperature on an empty stomach every day until the tapeworms are expelled. Be sure the tapeworms are intact as they are eliminated. If tapeworms are not eliminated intact, continue to eat *pepitas.*

Teeth

For strong and healthy teeth, chew on *cañaigre* root.

Teething

Cool a weak decoction of *comino* (cumin) tea, then give it to the teething baby. Add some sugar to sweeten its bitter taste.

Throat Infection

See Sore Throat

Thumb Sucking

To break a child's habit of thumb sucking, dip the thumb in hot saltwater.

Ticks

A surefire way to force a tick to release its grip is to burn it off with a lit cigarette or the hot tip of a blown-out match. Warning: Avoid direct contact with skin, as this may cause third degree burns.

Tonsillitis

Heat *plátano* (plantain banana) peels and spread butter on the inside of the peel. While they are still warm, place the peels on the throat, butter side down. Keep on for an hour.

Gargle with warm water that has a pinch of *chile* (cayenne pepper) in it. Always wash your hands after touching this spice. If you accidentally get some in your eyes, rinse with milk.

Mix lard and coffee grounds. Spread on banana peels, then use as a *plantilla* (foot poultice).

When tonsils swell, knead the arms with Vicks Vaporub. Some people believe that a sore throat causes knotting in the arms, so a deep kneading will release the balls of nerves. You'll feel better the next day.

Gargle with vinegar, salt, and warm water.

It is common in the countryside of Mexico to rub *baba*, or the foam that drips from the mouth of a horse, on the neck to help alleviate soreness from inflamed tonsils. This practice began when the Spanish first arrived. The Indians saw the horses with their extremely large necks and throats. They asked for the *baba*, thinking it would cure inflamed tonsils. This remedy has been passed down for about 500 years and apparently works.

Toothache

For fast relief, coat *clavos* (cloves) with olive oil or lard, then place them on the cavity.

Smash a clove of raw *ajo* (garlic) and place it directly onto the gum.

Place a pinch of *yerba del indio* (Indian root) and lard on the tooth, or rinse the mouth with a tincture made with the same plant.

Chew on *oshá* (lovage) root.

Tuberculosis

Drink boiled *zarzaparrilla* (sarsaparilla) root.

Tumors

To dissolve tumors under the skin, rub warm *aceite de almendras* (almond oil) on the sensitive area. If the tumor is growing inward, take 1 teaspoon oil twice a day, preferably on an empty stomach.

Make a poultice with arnica flowers and apply it to the skin tumor.

A good remedy for softening tumors is a poultice of the mashed *apio* (celery) plant. Apply a fresh poultice every evening.

Combine chopped *toloache* (jimson weed) and heated lard. Apply the poultice to the affected area. Wrap with gauze.

Crush a handful of green *llantén* (plantain) and mix with ½ cup olive oil. Apply the poultice on the affected area, then wrap with gauze or rags.

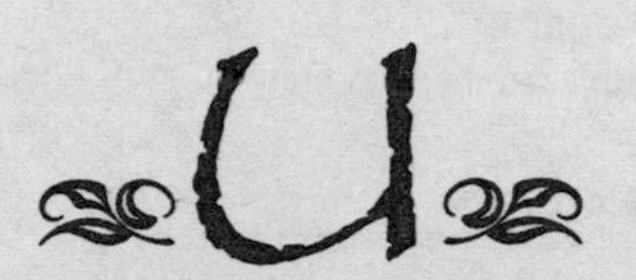

Si la píldora es muy grande,
es difícil tragarla.

If the pill is too large,
it is difficult to swallow.

Ulcers

Press and strain enough gel from the aloe vera plant to make 1 teaspoon aloe vera juice. Add the liquid to a glass of orange juice or water, and drink every morning before breakfast.

Drink a decoction of *apio* (celery) stems.

Make a tea with *plumajillo* (yarrow). Drink three times a day.

Drink 3 cups of *yerba mansa* (lizard tail) tea every day until you feel better.

Urinary Problems

See Kidney Disorders.

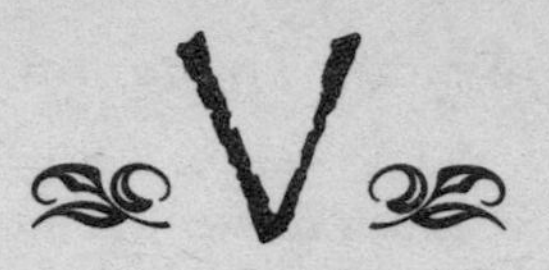

Dios le da pañuelos al que no tiene nariz.

God provides a hankerchief to those without a nose.

Vaginal Infection

For a good medicinal cleansing when you are suffering from a vaginal infection, nothing works as quickly as a douche. When making a douche decoction, use fresh rainwater when possible. Try any of the following herbs:

***Malva* (mallow) plant**
***Romero* (rosemary)**
***Rosa de Castilla* (rose) petals**
***Yerba del indio* (Indian root)**
***Yerba mansa* (lizard tail) leaves**

Varicose Veins

Elevate your feet on a pillow and drink a tea of alfalfa seeds two or three times a day until the swelling and pain ceases.

Cut an aloe vera leaf right down the middle, then heat the plant on a griddle. While it is still hot, rub the gel onto the varicose veins. Repeat as needed.

Make a tincture with arnica flowers and steep in a dark cupboard until the liquid changes color (a week or more). Strain and massage the liquid onto your calves and thighs, then prop your feet up on a pillow.

Drink a decoction of *apio* (celery) stems and lemon water daily, instead of tap water.

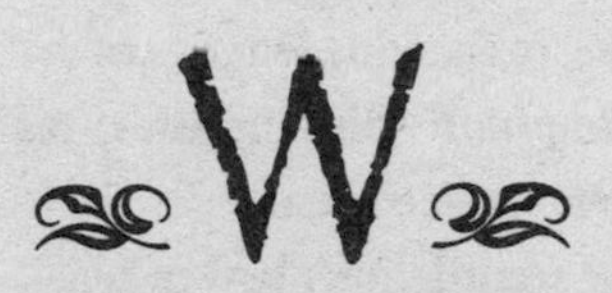

La esperanza muere al último.

Hope dies last of all.

WAKE UP

If you ever want to wake up at a certain time in the morning, you don't need an alarm clock. Merely tap one leg on the other. For example, if you want to get up at 6:00 A.M., just tap one leg on your other leg six times.

WARTS

For every wart that you have, tie a knot on a piece of string. Bury it in the backyard. As the string dissolves, the warts will go away.

WASH

The best way to clean your genitals is to bathe them with your own urine, about once a week or after sexual relations.

Drink a tea of *apio* (celery) stems and fresh lemon juice daily.

Water Retention

When your body withholds liquid, leaving you bloated, and you're incapable of buttoning your pants, choose from the following diuretics:

***Aguacate* (avocado) leaves tea**

***Aguja de piñon* (pine needles) tea**

***Apio* (celery) seed tea**

***Chicória* (dandelion) leaves tea**

***Flor de Santa Rita* (Indian paintbrush) tea**

***Flor saúco* (elder flowers) and berries tea**

Put crushed *nopal* (prickly-pear cactus) root and water in a glass jar, cover, and let steep in the hot sun all day. Drink the following morning.

Drink a decoction of *encino* (oak) bark.

Simmer *cabellos de elote fresco* (fresh corn silk) until the water turns dark brown. Drink 3 cups a day. It really works!

Weaning

To phase out breast milk, drink *albahaca* (basil) tea before nursing. This will reduce the flow of milk.

Once you have decided to wean your baby, start drinking *salvia* (sage) tea every day. This will dry up the milk.

Whooping Cough

Simmer *borraja* (borage) leaves and *canela* (cinnamon bark). Add honey. Sip as needed.

Drink a glass of hot *leche del burro* (donkey milk) simmered with a cinnamon stick.

Witchcraft (Protection Against)

Carry the root of the *oshá* (lovage) plant in your pocket or as an amulet, to avert the spells of *brujos* (witches).

Worms

To eliminate intestinal worms, make a decoction of the *aguacate* (avocado) skin and pit. Drink this hot liquid on an empty stomach. Be sure to plug your nose while you sip, so that the worms are not forewarned.

With the exception of tapeworms, *epazote* (wormseed tea) will rid the body of worms. Just simmer the seeds in milk, then drink.

Wounds

Always clean the wound well first. Apply cooked *col* (cabbage), at room temperature, directly on the wound, then wrap with gauze. Change the dressing and the *col* three times a day, for three days.

Apply a *maguey* (century plant) poultice on the wound.

To clean a wound, soak the area in a *consuelda* (comfrey) decoction, then cover with gauze.

Place a cold papaya poultice on the wound.

Apply a fresh *plumajillo* (yarrow) leaf poultice to the wound. This should stop the bleeding.

Chapter 4

Remedies at a Glance

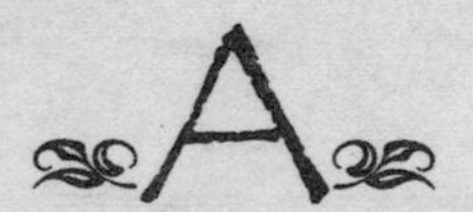

ALFALFA (*Medicago sativa*)

SPANISH: *alfalfa*

THERAPEUTIC USES: anemia, appetite stimulant, blood pressure, circulation, hangover, kidney disorders, stomachache, varicose veins

PARTS USED: sprouted seeds

APPLICATION:

TEA/INFUSION: 1 teaspoon dry or 2 teaspoons fresh alfalfa per cup of hot water. Steep for 10 minutes. Strain and sip 1 to 3 cups a day, for no more than 3 consecutive weeks. Sweeten to taste. Make fresh daily.

PROPERTIES: appetite stimulant, diuretic, laxative, tonic

WARNING: DO NOT TAKE IF YOU HAVE AN AUTOIMMUNE DISEASE. DO NOT EXCEED DOSAGE.

Originally from Asia and North Africa, this perennial plant's name comes from the Arabic word *alfasfasah*, meaning "the best fodder." Alfalfa is considered a good food source, since it readily releases nutrients. It contains chlorophyll, carotene, vitamins A, D, and K.

ALGAE

SPANISH: *lama del agua*

THERAPEUTIC USE: nosebleed

APPLICATION:
POULTICE: Skim the surface scum from a pond. Spread algae onto the back of the neck with your fingers. Cover with gauze or a towel. Make fresh as needed.

Algae varies in size, from single-celled forms to the giant kelp beds in the ocean. Though algae was at one time considered a plant, it is now classified separately. This is due to its lack of roots, stems, and leaves. Algae contains traces of calcium, phosphorus, sodium, and potassium.

ALMOND (*Prunus amygdalus*)

SPANISH: *almendra*
THERAPEUTIC USES: earache, tumors
PARTS USED: seed
APPLICATION:
OIL: Heat ½ cup olive oil in a double boiler. Add a handful of crushed almonds (9 or 10), then heat for an additional 30 minutes. Strain, then place a few drops in the ear while the oil is still warm. One-year shelf life.
PROPERTIES: demulcent, emollient

Indigenous to the Mediterranean, almond trees are also grown in California. Almond oil is used for perfumes, skin products, and medicine.

ALOE VERA (*Aloe vera*)

SPANISH: *aloe vera*
THERAPEUTIC USES: arthritis, athlete's foot, bruises, burns, constipation, cuts, eczema, hemorrhoids, insect bites, liver spots, ulcers, varicose veins
PART USED: leaves
APPLICATION:
INFUSION: Dissolve ¼ cup aloe vera gel in a tub of hot water, then soak.
POULTICE: Peel and extract ¼ cup fresh aloe vera gel. Heat gel and apply to the affected area. Cover with gauze or a towel. Make fresh daily.

TEA: Mix ½ teaspoon aloe vera gel in hot water. Sip ½ cup three times a day, for no more than two consecutive weeks. Make fresh daily.

TINCTURE: Add 1 part pounded aloe vera leaf to 3 parts alcohol and 2 parts water. Store in a dark, cool place for a week or two. Strain liquid into an airtight glass container. For external use only. Two-year shelf life.

PROPERTIES: anti-inflammatory, emollient, purgative

WARNING: DO NOT TAKE ALOE VERA INTERNALLY WHILE PREGNANT OR BREAST-FEEDING. DO NOT USE INTERNALLY IF YOU HAVE HEMORRHOIDS OR KIDNEY PROBLEMS.

Indigenous to Africa, the aloe vera plant has over 300 species. Aloe vera is a succulent resembling the cactus; Century plant is often mistaken for aloe vera, though the latter has more juice and less fiber. According to the Bible, aloe vera and myrrh were used in the embalming of Christ (John 19:39–40). The clear gel in aloe vera was one of Cleopatra's beauty secrets. This emollient contains aloectin B, which aids in the healing of minor burns and stopping infection. It is said that if an aloe vera plant is given as a gift, it will bring good luck to the house. Make a present of them, and hopefully one will be presented to you.

ANGELICA *(Angelica archangelica)*

SPANISH: *angélica*

THERAPEUTIC USES: bronchitis, colic, heartburn, stomachache

PARTS USED: roots, leaves

APPLICATION:

TEA/INFUSION: 1 teaspoon dry or 2 teaspoons fresh angelica roots or leaves per cup of hot water. Steep for 10 minutes. Strain and sip ½ cup three times a day, for no more than two consecutive weeks. Sweeten to taste. Make fresh daily.

TINCTURE: Add 1 part chopped angelica root to 3 parts alcohol (at least 80 proof) and 2 parts water. (Never use rubbing alcohol [isopropyl alcohol]; it is extremely toxic if taken internally.) Store in a dark, cool place for a week or two. Strain liquid into an airtight container. Take 20 drops. Two-year shelf life.

PROPERTIES: antispasmodic, carminative, diaphoretic, expectorant, stomachic, tonic

WARNING: DO NOT TAKE INTERNALLY WHILE PREGNANT OR WHILE BREASTFEEDING. DO NOT TAKE IF YOU ARE DIABETIC OR IF YOU HAVE RHEUMATISM OR NEURALGIA.

The ''angelic herb,'' as the name implies, comes from the medieval notion in Europe that the plant had holy powers against illness and witchcraft. This highly aromatic perennial plant soothes spasms, promotes perspiration, and acts as an anti-inflammatory. The volatile oil works as an expectorant by stimulating circulation.

ANISEED *(Pimpinella anisum)*

SPANISH: *anís*

THERAPEUTIC USES: colds, coughs, flatulence, indigestion, lactation, *mal de ojo*, menopause, pneumonia, stress, *susto*

PART USED: seeds

APPLICATION:

OINTMENT/SALVE: Slowly heat ⅓ to ½ cup lard or petroleum jelly in a double boiler over low heat. Add 2 or 3 tablespoons crushed aniseed, then heat for an additional hour. Strain and store in an airtight glass container. Two-year shelf life.

STEAM INHALATION: In a pot or old teakettle, simmer a strong infusion or decoction over low heat. Remove from heat source. Drape a towel over your head and inhale the steam.

TEA/INFUSION: 1 teaspoon crushed aniseed per cup of hot water. Steep for 10 minutes. Strain and sip when needed. Sweeten to taste. Make fresh daily.

TINCTURE: Add 1 part crushed aniseed to 3 parts alcohol (at least 80 proof). (Never use rubbing alcohol [isopropyl alcohol]; it is extremely toxic if taken internally.) Store in a dark, cool place for a week or two. Strain liquid into an airtight container. Take 20 drops in a glass of juice or water, two or three times a day. Two-year shelf life.

PROPERTIES: antiseptic, antispasmodic, aromatic, carminative, digestive, expectorant, stomachic, tonic

WARNING: DO NOT EXCEED INTERNAL DOSAGE WHILE PREGNANT OR WHILE BREASTFEEDING. THE ESSENTIAL OIL MAY BE TOXIC.

Native to Egypt and the Mediterranean region, this licorice-tasting herb has been of medicinal value for over 4,000 years. The Moors brought aniseed to the Spanish, who in turn shipped the plant to the Americas. Aniseed is an aromatic annual plant that aids the respiratory tract. It is often recommended for small children and infants. Aniseed can be found in a number of medicinal and culinary products.

ARNICA/LEOPARD'S BANE *(Arnica montana)*

SPANISH: *arnica*

THERAPEUTIC USES: aches, backaches, bruises, sprains, tumors, varicose veins

PARTS USED: flowers, rhizomes

APPLICATION:

OINTMENT/SALVE: Slowly heat ⅓ to ½ cup lard or petroleum jelly in a double boiler over low heat. Add 2 or 3 tablespoons crushed arnica flowers and roots, then heat for an additional hour. Strain and store in an airtight glass container. Two-year shelf life.

POULTICE: Crush and chop ½ to 1 cup fresh or dried arnica. Add enough hot water or oil to act as a binder. Dab olive oil on skin, then apply the poultice to the affected area. Cover with gauze or a towel. Make fresh daily.
TINCTURE: Add 1 part chopped arnica plant to 3 parts alcohol and 2 parts water. Store in a dark, cool place for a week or two. Strain liquid into an airtight glass container. For external use only. Two-year shelf life.

PROPERTIES: emollient

WARNING: FOR EXTERNAL USE ONLY. DO NOT USE IF SKIN IS IRRITATED OR DAMAGED. DO NOT USE WHILE PREGNANT OR WHILE BREASTFEEDING. IF RASH OCCURS, RINSE OFF SKIN IMMEDIATELY AND DISCONTINUE USE.

The name *arnica* comes from the ancient Greek word *arnakis*, or "lamb's skin," due to its supple petals. Arnica's medicinal uses were discovered separately by Native Americans and Europeans. Though toxic if taken internally, minute doses of arnica are prescribed by physicians for heart conditions.

ARTICHOKE *(Cynara scolymus)*

SPANISH: *alcachofa*
THERAPEUTIC USES: cirrhosis, diabetes
PARTS USED: leaves, roots
APPLICATION:

DECOCTION: In a saucepan add ⅛ cup pounded and crushed artichoke leaves per cup of cold water. Cover and simmer for 30 minutes or until liquid is reduced by ⅓. Strain and sip ½ cup of the decoction three times a day. Sweeten to taste. Make fresh daily.
POULTICE: Crush and chop ½ to 1 cup freshly pounded and chopped artichoke leaves and roots. Add enough hot water to act as a binder. Dab olive oil on skin, then apply

the poultice to the affected area. Cover with gauze or a towel. Make fresh daily.

PROPERTIES: cholagogue, diuretic, tonic

This perennial plant from the Mediterranean region was harvested by the Romans some 2,000 years ago. The name *artichoke* is derived from the Italian word *articiocco*, or "pine cone." Artichokes are a good source of vitamins A and C and are high in iron and calcium. Artichokes also contain cynarin, known for its curative effects on the liver.

ASH (*Fraxinus spp.*)

SPANISH: *fresno*

THERAPEUTIC USES: arthritis, fever

PART USED: leaves

APPLICATION:

TEA/INFUSION: ½ teaspoon dry or 1 teaspoon fresh ash leaves per cup of hot water. Steep for 10 minutes. Strain and sip ½ cup three times a day, for no more than two consecutive weeks. Sweeten to taste. Make fresh daily.

TINCTURE: Add 1 part chopped and bruised ash leaves to 3 parts alcohol (at least 80 proof) and 2 parts water. (Never use rubbing alcohol [isopropyl alcohol]; it is extremely toxic if taken internally.) Store in a dark cool place for a week or two. Strain liquid into an airtight container. Take 15 drops in a glass of juice or water two or three times a day. Two-year shelf life.

PROPERTIES: anti-inflammatory, astringent, diaphoretic, diuretic, tonic

Over 60 species of ash trees can be found growing throughout the world. The branches and leaves of this deciduous tree were once thought to act as a snake repellent.

ASPEN (*Populus tremuloides*)

SPANISH: *álamo*

THERAPEUTIC USES: fever, labor, sinus infection

PART USED: leaves, bark

APPLICATION:

DECOCTION: In a saucepan add 1 teaspoon dried and crushed or 3 teaspoons freshly chopped aspen bark and leaves per cup of cold water. Cover and simmer for 30 minutes or until liquid is reduced by ⅓. Strain and sip ½ cup of the decoction three or four times a day, for no more than one week. Sweeten to taste. Make fresh daily.

STEAM INHALATION: In a pot or old teakettle, simmer an infusion or decoction over low heat. Remove from heat source. Drape a towel over your head and inhale the steam.

PROPERTIES: antiseptic, astringent, anti-inflammatory, antipyretic, expectorant

WARNING: DO NOT USE IF ALLERGIC TO ASPIRIN. DO NOT EXCEED PRESCRIBED DOSAGE.

Indigenous to North America, this bitter tonic is not only a proven pain reliever, but a fever reducer as well. Similar to the willow, aspen contains salicin and salicylates; both derivatives are found in aspirin.

AVOCADO *(Persea americana)*

SPANISH: *aguacate*

THERAPEUTIC USES: aches, colic, dandruff, diabetes, diarrhea, gums, hair, menstrual cramps, rheumatism, skin care, spider bites, split ends, water retention, worms

PARTS USED: fruit, peel, pit, leaves, bark

APPLICATION:

TEA/INFUSION: 1 teaspoon dry or 2 teaspoons fresh avocado leaves per cup of hot water. Steep for 10 minutes. Strain and sip ½ cup three times a day. Sweeten to taste. Make fresh daily.

DECOCTION: In a saucepan add a crushed pit and chopped peel of 1 avocado to 3 cups cold water. Cover and simmer for 30 minutes or until liquid is reduced by ⅓. Strain and sip ½ cup of the decoction three times a day. Sweeten to taste. Make fresh daily.

POULTICE: Crush and chop an avocado pit. Add enough hot water to act as a binder. Dab olive oil on skin, then apply the poultice onto the affected area. Cover with gauze or a towel. Make fresh daily.

TINCTURE: Add 1 macerated avocado pit to 3 parts alcohol (at least 80 proof) and 2 parts water. Store in a dark, cool place until liquid turns a tea color. Strain liquid into an airtight glass container. For external use only. Two-year shelf life.

PROPERTIES: anthelmintic, astringent, carminative, diuretic, emmenagogue, emollient

Native to the Americas, some 400 varieties of this tree can be found throughout the world. Avocado was considered a panacea by Aztec, Incan, and Mayan mothers. Avocado contains 14 minerals and is a rich source of vitamin B as well as vitamins A and D. The oil from the pit or stone contains steroids and is noted for its antibiotic properties. Avocados are sugarless and have been proven to reduce cholesterol levels. Keep in mind that avocados are high in fat and calories.

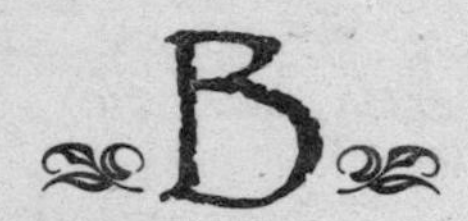

BANANA (*Musa paradisasa)*

SPANISH: *plátano*

THERAPEUTIC USE: tonsillitis

PART USED: peel

APPLICATION:

POULTICE: Heat peels on stovetop and spread butter on the insides of the peels. Dab olive oil on skin, then apply the poultice of hot peels, butter side down, to the affected area. Cover with a towel. Make fresh daily.

PROPERTY: astringent

Though not as popular in the United States as the sweet banana, this cooking plantain is often the accompaniment to traditional Latin American dishes. *Plantillas*, or poultices for the feet, are more common in Mexico than in the United States, and have been part of medicinal lore for centuries.

Basil (*Ocimum basilicum*)

Spanish: *albahacar, albahaca*

Therapeutic uses: appetite stimulant, colic, depression, earache, gas, labor, menstrual cramps, sore throat, *susto*, weaning

Parts used: leaves, flowers

Application:

tea/infusion: 2 teaspoons fresh basil leaves per cup of hot water. Steep for 10 minutes. Strain and sip ½ cup three times a day. Sweeten to taste. Make fresh daily.

Properties: analgesic, antibacterial, antispasmodic, carminative, emmenagogue, febrifuge, stomachic

Originally native to Asia, there are now 150 species of *Ocimum* growing throughout tropical and subtropical regions. It is said that this warm and spicy annual plant was discovered growing around the tomb of Christ after his resurrection. In Mexico, basil is often grown in front of houses and *yerberias* (herb stores) for protection. Sweet basil is one of the most popular species of basil, and is one of the most utilized medicinal herbs in Mexican kitchens. A sprig is sometimes carried for good fortune and love.

Bean (*various species*)

Spanish: *fríjol*

Therapeutic use: burns, canker sores, sunburn

Application:

poultice: Boil beans until soft and let cool. Mash ½ to 1 cup pinto beans, then apply the poultice to the affected area. Cover with a damp towel. Change dressing when paste begins to dry.

PROPERTY: antibiotic

There are at least 150 different species of beans found throughout the world, many of which have played a part in folklore and medicine. Bean meal has been used for skin problems for over a thousand years. Beans are a staple of the Mexican diet, and were part of the Aztecs' diet as well. The refried method of preparing beans surfaced after the Spanish arrival. Beans are an excellent source of fiber, protein, and starch, and may reduce cholesterol levels.

BORAGE *(Borago officianalis)*

SPANISH: *borraja*

THERAPEUTIC USES: bronchitis, eye irritation, fever, insomnia, mouthwash, whooping cough

PARTS USED: leaves, flowers, seeds

APPLICATION:

EYE WASH: Boil 1 cup of water and add 1 teaspoon finely chopped borage leaves and a dash of salt. Cool, then strain and use. Make fresh daily.

TEA/INFUSION: 1 teaspoon dry or 2 teaspoons fresh borage leaves and seeds per ½ cup of hot water. Steep for 5 minutes. Strain and sip ½ cup three times a day, for no more than two consecutive weeks. Sweeten to taste. Make fresh daily.

PROPERTIES: antidepressant, demulcent, diuretic, expectorant, febrifuge, tonic, sedative

WARNING: DO NOT TAKE IN LARGE DOSES OR ON A LONG-TERM BASIS, ESPECIALLY IF YOU HAVE A LIVER CONDITION. IF CONTACT DERMATITIS OCCURS, RINSE OFF SKIN IMMEDIATELY, AND DISCONTINUE USE.

The Moors referred to this annual plant, native to Syria, as "the father of sweat." Borage acts as a sedative and relieves tissue damage. The volatile oil balances hormonal activity and reduces blood pressure.

Bran

Spanish: *salvado*
Therapeutic uses: feet, pimples
Part used: corain
Application:
decoction: In a saucepan add 1 teaspoon dried and crushed bran to 1 cup of cold water. Cover and simmer for 30 minutes or until liquid is reduced by ⅓. Strain and use as a rinse. Make fresh daily.

Bran is the broken outer layers of grain, separated during the milling process. Approximately 25 percent of bran is fiber, making it an excellent source of dietary fiber.

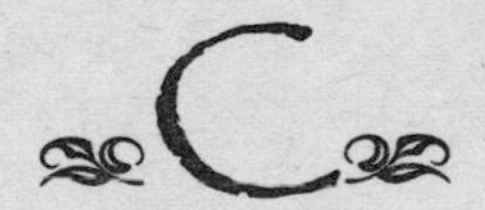

Cabbage (*Brassica oleracea*)

Spanish: *col*
Therapeutic uses: bee stings, wounds
Part used: leaves
Application:
poultice: Cut the midrib from several cabbage leaves and boil. Dab olive oil on skin, then apply the cooled leaves to the affected area. Cover with gauze or a towel. Change the dressing every few hours.
Properties: anti-inflammatory, antiseptic, vulnerary

Cabbage is an ancient vegetable that, according to myth, is the product of Zeus' perspiration. It is actually native to the Mediterranean region, where it has been cultivated for 4,000 years. When cabbage is applied to the skin, the sulfur in the leaves destroys bacteria, which can infect a puncture or cut. Cabbage is an excellent source of vitamins A, B, and C; potassium; and calcium. Cabbage is also a good source of roughage.

Camphor *(Cinnamomum camphora)*

Spanish: *alcanfor*

Therapeutic uses: aches, chicken pox, congestion, fever, headaches, measles

Parts used: leaves, stems, roots

Applications:

ointment/salve: Slowly heat ⅓ to ½ cup lard or petroleum jelly in a double boiler over low heat. Add 2 or 3 tablespoons finely chopped camphor leaves, then heat for an additional hour. Mix in 1 tablespoon baking soda. Strain and store in an airtight glass container. Two-year shelf life.

poultice: Crush and chop ½ to 1 cup fresh or dried camphor leaves. Add enough hot oil to act as a binder. Dab olive oil on skin, then apply the poultice to the affected area. Cover with gauze or a towel. Make fresh daily.

steam inhalation: In a pot or old teakettle, simmer an infusion or decoction of camphor leaves and stems over low heat. Remove from heat source. Drape a towel over your head and inhale the steam.

tincture: Add 1 part camphor plant to 3 parts alcohol, and 2 parts water. Store in a dark, cool place for a week or two. Strain liquid into an airtight glass container. For external use only. Two-year shelf life.

Properties: antiseptic, antispasmodic

WARNING: DO NOT TAKE INTERNALLY. BECAUSE THE EXTRACT IS EASILY ABSORBED BY THE SKIN TISSUES, IT MAY CAUSE NUMBNESS.

This evergreen tree is native to China, with over 250 species now grown worldwide. Camphor extracts are found in many over-the-counter products such as Ben-Gay and Vicks Vaporub. Camphor oil is an effective ointment due to its ability to be absorbed quickly into the skin.

CANAIGRE (*Rumex hymenosepalus*)

SPANISH: *cañaigre*
THERAPEUTIC USES: sore throat, teeth
PARTS USED: root
APPLICATION:

DECOCTION: In a saucepan add 1 teaspoon dried or 3 teaspoons fresh, chopped canaigre root per cup of cold water. Cover and simmer for 30 minutes or until liquid is reduced by ⅓. Strain and sip ½ cup of the decoction three times a day. Sweeten to taste. Make fresh daily.

PROPERTIES: astringent, hemostatic.

Canaigre is native to the southwestern United States and northern Mexico. The leaves contain vitamins A and C and can be prepared like spinach.

CASCARA SAGRADA (*Rhamnus purshiana*)

SPANISH: *cáscara sagrada*
THERAPEUTIC USES: constipation, stomachache
PART USED: bark
APPLICATION:

DECOCTION: In a saucepan add 1 teaspoon dried bark per 2 cups cold water. Cover and simmer for 30 minutes or until liquid is reduced by ⅓. Strain and sip 1 cup of the cold decoction before going to bed. Sweeten to taste. Make fresh daily.

WARNING: DO NOT USE IF YOU HAVE BOWEL DISEASES OR ULCERS. DISCONTINUE USE IF NAUSEA OCCURS. DO NOT USE OVER A LONG PERIOD OF TIME.

PROPERTIES: antispasmodic, purgative, tonic

The early Mexican priests dubbed this native tree ''the sacred bark,'' after discovering its use as a gentle laxative. It is non–habit forming and is found in most over-the-counter laxatives.

CATCLAW (*Acacia greggii*)

SPANISH: *uña de gato*

THERAPEUTIC USES: aches, bruises, hangover, headache, nerves, stomachache

PARTS USED: pods, leaves

APPLICATION:

TINCTURE: Add 1 part bruised catclaw pods and leaves to 3 parts alcohol (at least 80 proof) and 2 parts water. (Never use rubbing alcohol [isopropyl alcohol]; it is extremely toxic if taken internally.) Store in a dark, cool place for a week or two. Strain liquid into an airtight glass container. Two-year shelf life.

PROPERTIES: antibiotic, astringent, emollient, stomachic

This small shrub has thorns similar to a rose or the claw of a cat. Catclaw is from the Peruvian rainforest and is used for stimulating the immune system.

CAYENNE PEPPER (*Capsicum frutescens*)

SPANISH: *chile*

THERAPEUTIC USES: colds, earache, tonsillitis

PART USED: entire pepper, dried and ground into powder

APPLICATION:

OIL: Heat ½ cup olive oil in a double boiler. Add ½ tablespoon cayenne pepper, then heat for an additional 20 minutes. Pour warm liquid into an ear dropper. One-year shelf life.

TEA/INFUSION: ½ teaspoon dry cayenne pepper per cup of hot water. Steep for 10 minutes. Strain and sip ½ cup three times a day, for no more than two consecutive weeks. Make fresh daily.

PROPERTIES: analgesic, antiseptic, astringent, diaphoretic, digestive, stimulant

WARNING: DO NOT TAKE WHILE PREGNANT OR BREASTFEEDING. DO NOT TAKE

IF YOU HAVE ULCERS. IF CONTACT DERMATITIS OCCURS, RINSE OFF IMMEDIATELY AND DISCONTINUE USE.

This perennial plant is indigenous to Mexico, South America, and Zanzibar. Its genus name, *Capsicum*, is Greek for "to bite." There are several hundred domesticated species of *Capsicum* growing in all parts of the tropics. Cayenne promotes sweating, stimulates circulation, and invigorates the heart. Capsaicin, a derivative of the seeds, may contain antibiotic properties. The volatile oil may cause irritation.

CELERY (*Apium graveolens*)

SPANISH: *apio*

THERAPEUTIC USES: nerves, stomachache, tumors, ulcers, varicose veins, water retention

PARTS USED: root, leaves, seeds

APPLICATION:

DECOCTION: In a saucepan add 1 teaspoon freshly chopped celery stalks and seeds per cup of cold water. Cover and simmer for 5 minutes. Strain and sip ½ cup of the decoction twice a day. Sweeten to taste. Make fresh daily.

POULTICE: Crush and chop ½ to 1 cup freshly chopped celery stalks. Add enough hot water or oil to act as a binder. Dab olive oil on skin, then apply the poultice to the affected area. Cover with gauze or a towel. Make fresh daily.

PROPERTIES: anti-inflammatory, antiseptic, antispasmodic, carminative, diuretic, emmenagogue, sedative, tonic

WARNING: DO NOT EXCEED PRESCRIBED DOSAGE FOR INTERNAL USE WHILE PREG-

NANT OR BREASTFEEDING. DO NOT USE INTERNALLY IF YOU HAVE ACUTE KIDNEY DYSFUNCTION.

Historically, victors of early Greek sporting events were rewarded with this source of roughage. This biennial plant has also been of medicinal value for thousands of years.

CENTURY PLANT (*Agave spp.*)

SPANISH: *maguey*

THERAPEUTIC USES: abscesses, constipation, diabetes, wounds

PARTS USED: fiber, sap

APPLICATION:

POULTICE: Crush and chop ½ cup fresh century plant fiber and sap. Apply the poultice to the affected area. Cover with gauze or a towel. Make fresh daily.

TEA/INFUSION: 1 teaspoon dry or 2 teaspoons fresh century plant sap per cup of hot water. Sip ½ cup three times a day, hot or cold. Sweeten to taste. Make fresh daily.

PROPERTIES: anti-inflammatory, antiseptic, demulcent, diaphoretic, laxative

WARNING: DO NOT TAKE INTERNALLY WHILE PREGNANT OR BREASTFEEDING. EXCESSIVE USE MAY CAUSE LIVER DAMAGE.

This succulent is indigenous to Central America. The name *century plant* derives from the folk belief that the plant would bloom every hundred years. Century plant is an important resource among the desert regions of Mexico. The leaves supply food, drink, soap, rope, and shingled rooftops. Tequila, mescal, and pulque are distilled liquors made from the sap of this plant. Century plant contains vitamins A, B, C, D, and K.

CHAMOMILE (*Matricaria chamomilla*)

SPANISH: *manzanilla*

THERAPEUTIC USES: colds, colic, congestion, cramps, earache, eczema, eye inflammation, flu, hair, insomnia, kidney disorders, labor, miscarriage, stomachache

PARTS USED: flowers, leaves

APPLICATION:

OIL: Heat ½ cup olive oil in a double boiler. Add 3 tablespoons crushed chamomile plant, then heat for an additional 20 minutes. Strain warm liquid into an airtight glass container. One-year shelf life.

POULTICE: Crush and chop ½ to 1 cup fresh or dried chamomile plant. Add enough hot water or oil to act as a binder. Dab olive oil on skin, then apply the poultice to the affected area. Cover with gauze or a towel. Make fresh daily.

STEAM INHALATION: In a pot or old teakettle, simmer a strong infusion or decoction over low heat. Remove from heat source. Drape a towel over your head and inhale the steam.

TEA/INFUSION: 1 teaspoon dry or 2 teaspoons fresh chamomile flowers per cup of hot water. Steep for 10 minutes. Strain and sip ½ cup three times a day. Make fresh daily.

TINCTURE: Add 1 part chamomile flowers and leaves to 3 parts alcohol (at least 80 proof) and 2 parts water. (Never use rubbing alcohol [isopropyl alcohol]; it is extremely toxic if taken internally.) Store in a dark, cool place for a week or two. Strain liquid into an airtight glass container. Take 10 to 15 drops in a glass of water, two or three times a day. Two-year shelf life.

PROPERTIES: anodyne, antibacterial, anti-inflammatory, antispasmodic, calmative, carminative, tonic

The Greek name for chamomile is *kamai*, "on the ground," or *melon*, "little apple," because of the applelike scent from the leaves. This annual plant is another of the universally recognized folk medicines. Chamomile has been proven to alleviate pain and promote healing.

CHAPARRAL/CREOSOTE BUSH *(Larrea tridentata)*

SPANISH: *hediondilla, gobernadora*

THERAPEUTIC USES: arthritis, blood pressure, headache, kidney disorders, pimples, respiratory problems, skin cancer

PARTS USED: leaves, branches

APPLICATION:

DECOCTION: In a saucepan add 1 teaspoon of the young branches of the chaparral bush per cup of cold water. Cover and simmer for 30 minutes or until liquid is reduced by ⅓. Strain and sip ½ cup of the decoction three times a day. Sweeten to taste. Make fresh daily.

OIL: Heat ½ cup olive oil in a double boiler. Add 3 tablespoons of crushed chaparral leaves, then heat for an additional 20 minutes. Strain warm liquid into an airtight glass container. One-year shelf life.

POULTICE: Crush and chop ½ to 1 cup fresh or dried chaparral leaves. Add enough hot water or oil to act as a binder. Dab olive oil on skin, then apply the poultice to the affected area. Cover with gauze or a towel. Make fresh daily.

STEAM INHALATION: In a pot or old teakettle, simmer a strong infusion or decoction over low heat. Remove from heat source. Drape a towel over your head and inhale the steam.

TEA/INFUSION: 1 teaspoon dry or 2 teaspoons fresh chaparral leaves per cup of hot water. Steep for 10 minutes. Strain and sip ½ cup three times a day. Sweeten to taste. Make fresh daily.

PROPERTIES: antibiotic, astringent, diuretic

WARNING: DUE TO THE CONCERN OF HEPATITIS, THE SALE OF CHAPARRAL HAS RECENTLY BEEN BANNED IN THE UNITED STATES.

Indigenous to the desert regions, chaparral was considered a *sanalotodo* (cure-all) by northern Mexicans and people in the southern United States. Chaparral is one of the best natural antibiotics, but contains nordihydroguairetic acid, which is harmful to the liver.

CHICKEN DROPPINGS

THERAPEUTIC USE: *empacho*

Wild birds were part of ceremony and sustenance for the Indian people long before Spain introduced the chicken to Mexico. Animal parts and excrement are still featured in the ritual practices, surviving the Spanish conquest and assimilation into the U.S.

CHOCOLATE *(Cocoa)*

SPANISH: *chocolate*
THERAPEUTIC USE: headache
PART USED: seeds

Chocolate was without a doubt the best received export from the New World. Even the name ''chocolate'' escaped translation, and is still similar to Nahuatl's, *Chocólatl.* The beans were used as currency by the Incas, Mayans, and Aztecs. Chocolate is made from the seeds of the theobroma tree, and contains caffeine which acts as a stimulant.

Cocoa powder has nervine and stimulant properties, and is used to lower blood pressure.

CINNAMON *(Cinnamomum zeylanicum)*

SPANISH: *canela*
THERAPEUTIC USES: *aire, bilis*, colds, cramps, fever,

hangover, morning sickness, nausea, postpartum care, stomachache, *susto,* whooping cough

PART USED: bark

APPLICATION:

DECOCTION: Pound and bruise 1 tablespoon cinnamon bark per cup of cold water. Simmer until liquid turns amber, about 10 minutes. Strain and sip ½ cup of the decoction three times a day. Sweeten to taste. Make fresh daily.

PROPERTIES: antirheumatic, antiseptic, antispasmodic, antiviral, carminative, emmenagogue, sedative, stomachic, tonic

Indigenous to Sri Lanka, cinnamon bark has been of medicinal use for over 3,000 years. This warm and woody spice was used by the Egyptians in the practice of embalming. Cinnamon is the oldest spice referred to in the Bible; it was an ingredient in the holy anointing oil of Moses (Exodus 30:23).

CLOVE (*Eugenia caryophyllata*)

SPANISH: *clavo*

THERAPEUTIC USES: bronchitis, cramps, earache, hangover, nausea, toothache

PART USED: flower buds

APPLICATION:

DECOCTION: In a saucepan add 1 teaspoon dried and crushed cloves per cup of cold water. Cover and simmer for 30 minutes or until liquid is reduced by ⅓. Strain and sip ½ cup of the decoction three times a day. Sweeten to taste. Make fresh daily.

OIL: Heat ½ cup olive oil in a double boiler. Add 3 tablespoons crushed cloves, then heat for an additional 20 minutes. Strain warm liquid into an airtight glass container. One-year shelf life.

PROPERTIES: analgesic, antiseptic, antispasmodic, carminative, expectorant

WARNING: DO NOT SUBSTITUTE CLOVE OIL CONCENTRATE FOR THIS REMEDY. IT IS EXTREMELY PAINFUL. IF CONTACT DERMATITIS OCCURS, RINSE OFF SKIN IMMEDIATELY AND DISCONTINUE USE.

Indigenous to Indonesia, this aromatic spice is considered a cure-all in Southeast Asia. Over 450 species can be found growing throughout the tropical world. The pink flowers are plucked, becoming spicy and warm as they dry. Some cultures believe that cloves are an aphrodisiac.

COFFEE *(Coffea spp.)*

SPANISH: *café*
THERAPEUTIC USE: headache, nausea, tonsillitis
PART USED: seeds
APPLICATION:
POULTICE: Crush ½ to 1 cup coffee beans. Add enough hot lard to act as a binder. Spread on the inner peel of a banana. Dab olive oil on skin before applying the poultice to the affected area. Change poultice as needed or every few hours.
PROPERTIES: digestive, diuretic, stimulant

WARNING: DO NOT TAKE IF YOU HAVE HIGH BLOOD PRESSURE OR HEART PALPITATIONS.

Coffee is indigenous to East Africa, but now many of the 40 species can be found in most tropical regions. Coffee has been used in the treatment of nausea in homeopathic medicine for centuries. Almost ⅓ of the coffee bean is the stimulant caffeine.

COMFREY *(Symphytum officinale)*

SPANISH: *consuelda*
THERAPEUTIC USES: broken bones, bronchitis, bruises, menstrual flow, pimples, psoriasis, wounds

PARTS USED: leaves, root

APPLICATION:

DECOCTION: In a saucepan add 1 teaspoon dried or 3 teaspoons chopped fresh comfrey roots per cup of cold water. Cover and simmer for 30 minutes or until liquid is reduced by ⅓. Strain and sip ½ cup of the decoction three times a day. Sweeten to taste. Make fresh daily.

OINTMENT/SALVE: Slowly heat ⅓ to ½ cup lard or petroleum jelly in a double boiler over low heat. Add 2 or 3 tablespoons finely chopped comfrey root, then heat for an additional hour. Strain and store in an airtight glass jar. Two-year shelf life.

POULTICE: Crush and chop ½ to 1 cup fresh or dried comfrey plant. Add enough hot water or oil to act as a binder. Dab olive oil on skin, then apply the poultice to the affected area. Cover with gauze or a towel. Make fresh daily.

TINCTURE: Add 1 part bruised comfrey root to 3 parts alcohol (at least 80 proof) and 2 parts water. (Never use rubbing alcohol [isopropyl alcohol]; it is extremely toxic if taken internally.) Store in a dark, cool place for a week or two. Strain liquid into an airtight glass container. Two-year shelf life.

WARNING: DO NOT TAKE INTERNALLY WHILE PREGNANT OR BREASTFEEDING. DO NOT EXCEED PRESCRIBED DOSAGE FOR INTERNAL USE. COMFREY CONTAINS PYRROLIZIDINE ALKALOIDS, A SUBSTANCE TOXIC TO THE LIVER.

PROPERTIES: anodyne, anti-inflammatory, astringent, expectorant, hemostatic, vulnerary

Throughout history, this perennial plant has been used to mend bones. *Conferva* is a Latin word meaning "grow together," while the genus name, *Symphytum*, comes to us from the Greek words *sympho*, "make it grow," and *phyton*, "plant."

This revered plant promotes cell proliferation, which

heals damaged tissue, and reduces inflammation. It was once believed that a comfrey bath would restore one's virginity.

CORIANDER (*Coriandrum sativum*)

SPANISH: *cilantro*
THERAPEUTIC USES: *aire*, cramps, gums, nerves
PARTS USED: leaves, seeds
APPLICATION:
TEA/INFUSION: 1 or 2 teaspoons of dried and crushed coriander seeds per cup of hot water. Steep for 10 minutes. Strain and sip ½ cup three times a day, for no more than two consecutive weeks. Add honey to taste. Make fresh daily.
DECOCTION: In a saucepan add 2 teaspoons dried and crushed coriander seeds per cup of cold water. Cover and simmer for 30 minutes or until liquid is reduced by ⅓. Strain and sip ½ cup of the decoction three times a day. Sweeten to taste. Make fresh daily.
PROPERTIES: antispasmodic, appetite stimulant, aromatic, carminative, nervine, stomachic

The two species of this annual are native to Asia and Africa. Coriander has been used since ancient times; the Egyptians considered it an aphrodisiac. Its name derives from the Greek word *koriannon*, a bedbug which gave off the scent of the herb. Coriander was one of the first spices to be cultivated in America. Coriander leaves, or cilantro, are a standard ingredient in Mexican salsas and dishes. Coriander contains volatile oil, which acts as a digestive aid.

CORNMEAL (*Zea mays*)

SPANISH: *masa*
THERAPEUTIC USES: boils, hangover, infections, stomachache
APPLICATION:
POULTICE: Mix cornmeal and enough hot water to make a dough. Dab olive oil on skin, then apply the poultice

to the affected area. Cover with gauze or a towel. Make fresh daily.

Corn has been grown in Mexico and Guatemala for over 3,000 years. Earthen vessels adorned with corn have been excavated from prehistoric sites in the highlands of Mexico. The Aztecs utilized corn for food, currency, and fashion. The botanical name *Zea* is Latin for "cause of life," and *maize* means "our mother." This annual is often sited as the most significant contribution of the New World. Corn is a complex carbohydrate, is relatively low in fat, and contains fiber.

CORN SILK *(Zea mays)*

SPANISH: *cabellos de elote*

THERAPEUTIC USES: *bilis,* burning urination, *espanto*, kidney disorders, water retention

APPLICATION:

TEA/INFUSION: 1 teaspoon dry or 2 teaspoons fresh corn silk per cup of hot water. Steep for 10 minutes. Strain and sip ½ cup three times a day. Make fresh daily.

PROPERTIES: antispasmodic, demulcent, diuretic

Corn silk is rich in potassium, which brings about urination, and eliminates bile flow. It is also able to break down and flush gravel from the bladder and kidneys.

CUMIN *(Cuminum cyminum)*

SPANISH: *comino*

THERAPEUTIC USES: digestion, flatulence, labor, teething

PART USED: seeds

APPLICATION:

DECOCTION: In a saucepan add 1 teaspoon dried and crushed cumin seeds per cup of cold water. Cover and simmer for 10 minutes. Strain and sip ½ cup of the decoction three times a day. Sweeten to taste. Make fresh daily.

PROPERTIES: anesthetic, carminative, digestive

This annual plant is native to Egypt, where it has been utilized to treat indigestion for centuries.

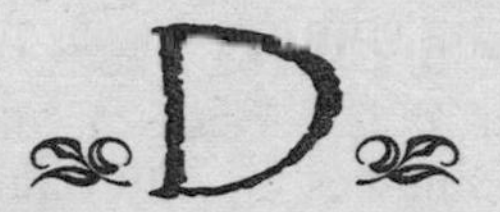

DAMIANA (*Turnera spp.*)

SPANISH: *damiana*

THERAPEUTIC USES: aphrodisiac, depression, diabetes, *frío en la matriz*, impotence

PART USED: leaves

APPLICATION:

TEA/INFUSION: 1 teaspoon dry or 2 teaspoons fresh damiana leaves per cup of hot water. Steep for 10 minutes. Strain and sip 2 cups a day, for no more than three consecutive weeks. Sweeten to taste. Make fresh daily.

TINCTURE: Add 1 part bruised and chopped damiana leaves to 3 parts alcohol (at least 80 proof) and 2 parts water. (Never use rubbing alcohol [isopropyl alcohol]; it is extremely toxic if taken internally.) Store in a dark, cool place for a week or two. Strain liquid into an airtight container. Take 1 teaspoon in a glass of juice or water. Two-year shelf life.

PROPERTIES: antidepressant, diuretic, laxative, tonic, stimulant

WARNING: DO NOT TAKE INTERNALLY WHILE PREGNANT, WHILE BREASTFEEDING OR DURING MENSTRUATION.

Indigenous to the Gulf of Mexico, damiana has long been used as an aphrodisiac by the Mayan and Aztec people (though this property has been neither proved nor disproved).

DANDELION (*Taraxacum officinale*)

SPANISH: *chicória, diente de león*

THERAPEUTIC USES: blood tonic, constipation, kidney stones, liver disorders, water retention

PART USED: whole plant

APPLICATION:

DECOCTION: In a saucepan add 1 teaspoon chopped fresh dandelion roots per cup of cold water. Cover and simmer for 30 minutes or until liquid is reduced by ⅓. Strain and sip ½ cup (hot or cold) of the decoction three times a day. Sweeten to taste. Make fresh daily.

TEA/INFUSION: 1 teaspoon dry or 2 teaspoons fresh dandelion leaves per cup of hot water. Steep for 10 minutes. Strain and sip 3 cups (hot or cold) a day. Sweeten to taste. Make fresh daily.

PROPERTIES: aperient, astringent, diuretic, stomachic, tonic

The leaves of this perennial plant are also a food source, and contain potassium and iron. The leaves revitalize liver function, and is an abundant source of vitamins A and C.

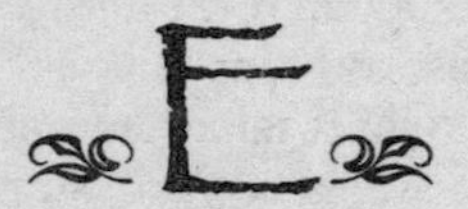

EGG

SPANISH: *huevo*

THERAPEUTIC USE: burns, calcium deficiency

SUPERNATURAL USE: evil eye, speed

PARTS USED: whole egg

Eggs have been part of folklore for centuries. They are symbolic of the soul, and are believed to maintain superstitious and therapeutic properties. The cool egg white is a familiar remedy for burns in a number of cultures.

Though eggs are a high source of protein and fat, a number of the medicinal uses are external. Eggs also contain vitamins A, B, C, D, E, as well as calcium and minerals.

ELDER (*Sambucus spp.*)

SPANISH: *saúco*

THERAPEUTIC USES: acne, *bilis*, blood pressure, chicken pox, colic, fever, heart tonic, heatstroke, hemorrhoids, measles, pimples, water retention

PARTS USED: leaves, flowers, bark

APPLICATION:

DECOCTION: In a saucepan add 1 teaspoon dried and crushed or 3 teaspoons chopped fresh elder bark per cup of cold water. Cover and simmer for 30 minutes or until liquid is reduced by ⅓. Strain and sip ½ cup of the decoction three times a day. Sweeten to taste. Make fresh daily.

OIL: Heat ½ cup olive oil in a double boiler. Add 3 tablespoons crushed elder leaves, then heat for an additional 20 minutes. Strain warm liquid into an airtight glass container. One-year shelf life.

TEA/INFUSION: 1 teaspoon dry or 2 teaspoons fresh elder leaves and/or flowers per cup of hot water. Steep for 10 minutes. Strain and sip ½ cup three times a day, for no more than two consecutive weeks. Sweeten to taste. Make fresh daily.

PROPERTIES: anti-inflammatory, carminative, diaphoretic, diuretic, expectorant, and stimulant

This deciduous tree grows on most of the continents. Elder holds the distinction of being one of the first plants documented for medicinal use some 1,700 years ago in Egypt.

EUCALYPTUS (*Eucaliptus spp.*)

SPANISH: *eucalipto*

THERAPEUTIC USES: asthma, bronchitis, colds, fever, flu

PARTS USED: leaves

APPLICATION:

STEAM INHALATION: In a pot or old teakettle, simmer a strong infusion of eucalyptus over low heat. Remove from heat source. Drape a towel over your head and inhale the steam.

TEA/INFUSION: 1 teaspoon dry or 2 teaspoons fresh eucalyptus leaves per cup of hot water. Steep for 10 minutes. Strain and sip ½ cup three times a day, for no more than two consecutive weeks. Sweeten to taste. Make fresh daily.

PROPERTIES: antiseptic, decongestant, diaphoretic, expectorant, stimulant

WARNING: DO NOT EXCEED PRESCRIBED DOSAGE FOR INTERNAL USE. THE ESSENTIAL OIL'S TOXICITY VARIES WITH EACH SPECIES.

Native to Australia and Tasmania, this evergreen has the distinction of being one of the fastest-growing trees in the world. Eucalyptus roots absorb massive amounts of water. For this reason, eucalyptus has been planted in marshy regions throughout the world, in successful attempts to dry up disease-infested water. The leaves of the eucalyptus tree contain essential oils that kill several types of bacteria and are an efficacious decongestant. Eucalyptus oil is now found in a variety of over-the-counter medicines.

EVENING PRIMROSE *(Oenothera biennis)*

SPANISH: *flor de San Juan*

THERAPEUTIC USES: eczema, freckles, kidney disorders, sore throat

PARTS USED: whole plant

APPLICATION:

OIL: Heat ½ cup olive oil in a double boiler. Add 3 tablespoons crushed evening primrose plant, then heat for an additional 20 minutes. Strain warm liquid into an airtight glass container. One-year shelf life.

POULTICE: Crush and chop ½ to 1 cup fresh or dried evening primrose plant. Add enough hot water or oil to act as a binder. Dab olive oil on skin, then apply the poultice to the affected area. Cover with gauze or a towel. Make fresh daily.

TEA/INFUSIONS: 1 teaspoon dry or 2 teaspoons fresh evening primrose flowers and leaves per cup of hot water. Steep for 10 minutes. Strain and sip ½ cup three times a day. Sweeten to taste. Make fresh daily.

PROPERTIES: astringent, sedative

WARNING: DO NOT TAKE INTERNALLY IF YOU HAVE EPILEPSY.

In order to pollinate, the evening primrose blooms at dusk and emanates a fragrance and phosphorescent light that attracts the nocturnal sphinx moth. Native to North America, this annual or biennial is high in fatty acids and contains gamma-linolenic acid, which acts as a catalyst in producing substances similar to hormones.

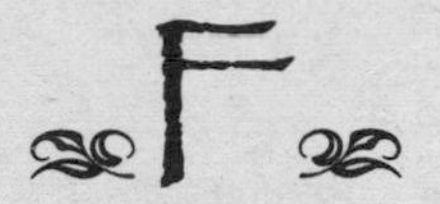

FENNEL (*Foeniculum vulgare*)

SPANISH: *hinojo*

THERAPEUTIC USES: appetite stimulant, colic, cramps, flatulence, lactation, migraines

PART USED: seeds

APPLICATION:

DECOCTION: In a saucepan add 1 teaspoon crushed fennel seeds per cup of cold water. Cover and simmer for 15 minutes. Strain and sip ½ cup of the decoction three times a day. Sweeten to taste. Make fresh daily.

STEAM INHALATION: In a pot or old teakettle, simmer a strong infusion or decoction of fennel over low heat. Remove from heat source. Drape a towel over your head and inhale the steam.

PROPERTIES: anti-inflammatory, antispasmodic, carminative, diuretic, expectorant, stimulant, stomachic

WARNING: DO NOT EXCEED PRESCRIBED DOSAGE FOR INTERNAL USE.

For over a thousand years, this aromatic perennial has been used as a spice and in medicine. Though fennel is native to the Mediterranean, Spanish priests were the first to introduce fennel to the Americas. In medieval times, fennel seeds were chewed during Lent. Fennel has similar folk uses to aniseed and caraway. The seeds contain volatile oil, which may produce a direct stimulant effect on the respiratory tract.

FLAXSEED *(Linum usitatissimum)*

SPANISH: *grano de lino*

THERAPEUTIC USES: constipation, kidney disorders, rheumatism

PARTS USED: seeds, oil

APPLICATION:

DECOCTION: In a saucepan add 1 teaspoon crushed flaxseed per cup of cold water. Cover and simmer for 20 minutes. Strain and sip ½ cup of the decoction three times a day, for no more than two consecutive weeks. Sweeten to taste. Make fresh daily.

OIL: Heat ½ cup olive oil in a double boiler. Add 3 tablespoons crushed flaxseed, then heat for an additional 20 minutes. Strain warm liquid into an airtight glass container. One-year shelf life.

PROPERTIES: anti-inflammatory, demulcent, emollient, purgative

WARNING: DO NOT INGEST IMMATURE SEED PODS, AS THEY MAY BE TOXIC. DO NOT CONSUME OVER A LONG PERIOD OF TIME.

Humankind has been familiar with this multifaceted plant for over 7,000 years. The Egyptian pharaohs were wrapped in the fiber of flax. Its early uses included clothing, food, and medicine. Linseed oil is derived from this annual plant.

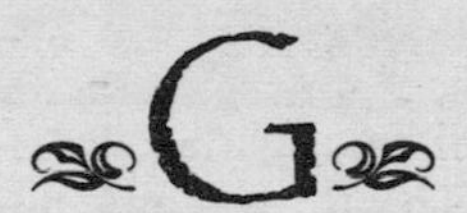

GARLIC *(allium sativum)*

SPANISH: *ajo*

THERAPEUTIC USES: acne, blood pressure, bronchitis, corns, cuts, earache, insect bites, insect repellent, nails, toothache

PART USED: bulb

APPLICATION:

DECOCTION: In a saucepan add 1 teaspoon crushed garlic cloves per cup of cold water. Cover and simmer for 30 minutes or until liquid is reduced by ⅓. Strain and sip ½ cup of the decoction three times a day. Sweeten to taste. Make fresh daily.

OIL: Heat ½ cup olive oil in a double boiler. Add 3 tablespoons crushed garlic, then heat for an additional 20 minutes. Strain warm liquid into an airtight glass container. One-year shelf life.

POULTICE: Crush and chop ½ to 1 cup fresh garlic cloves. Add enough hot water or oil to act as a binder. Dab olive oil on skin, then apply the poultice onto the affected area. Cover with gauze or a towel. Make fresh daily.

TINCTURE: Add 1 part pounded garlic to 3 parts alcohol (at least 80 proof) and 2 parts water. (Never use rubbing alcohol [isopropyl alcohol]; it is extremely toxic if taken internally.) Store in a dark, cool place for a week or two. Strain liquid into an airtight glass container. Take 20 drops in a glass of juice or water, two or three times a day. Two-year shelf life.

PROPERTIES: antibacterial, antibiotic, antifungal, antispasmodic, carminative, cholagogue, diuretic, expectorant, febrifuge, stimulant

WARNING: INTERNAL USE NOT RECOMMENDED FOR INFANTS.

Indigenous to Siberia, garlic was a favorite food of the ancient Israelites. The Bible states that while crossing the desert, the Israelites craved garlic and other foods (Numbers 11:4–6). Garlic is probably one of the most universally recognized plants in folk medicine. Though garlic has long been associated with the onion, this bulbous root is actually from the lily family. This favorite food, medicine, and charm has been utilized for centuries by the Old and New World. Garlic contains allicin, a powerful antibiotic equivalent to 1 percent of penicillin; vitamins A, C, and E; thiamine; and riboflavin.

GINGER *(Zingiber officinale)*

SPANISH: *ajengibre, jengibre*

THERAPEUTIC USES: feet, fever, hangover, indigestion, morning sickness, nausea, sinus infection, stomachache

PART USED: fresh rhizome

APPLICATION:

DECOCTION: In a saucepan add 1 teaspoon crushed or grated ginger root per cup of cold water. Cover and simmer for 20 minutes. Strain and sip ½ cup of the decoction three times a day. Sweeten to taste. Make fresh daily.

PROPERTIES: carminative, diaphoretic, stimulant

WARNING: DO NOT TAKE INTERNALLY IF YOU HAVE ULCERS.

According to European legend, ginger came from the Garden of Eden. Actually, this perennial plant is indigenous to Asia, where it has been used as a cure-all for at least 2,000 years.

GUAVA (*Psidium guajava*)

SPANISH: *guayaba*

THERAPEUTIC USES: amoebas, diarrhea

PARTS USED: fruit, leaves

APPLICATION:

TEA/INFUSION: 1 teaspoon dry or 2 teaspoons fresh guava leaves per cup of hot water. Steep for 10 minutes. Strain and sip ½ cup three times a day. Make fresh daily.

Indigenous to Central America, guavas were used for treating tissue damage by the Aztecs. The fruit is a rich source of vitamin C. Guavas also contain potassium, sulfur, and chlorine.

H

HOREHOUND (*Marrubium vulgare*)

SPANISH: *marrubio*

THERAPEUTIC USES: appetite stimulant, asthma, bronchitis, colic, *coraje*, coughs, *espanto*, frostbite, stomachache, *susto*

PART USED: leaves

APPLICATION:

TEA/INFUSION: 1 teaspoon dry or 2 teaspoons fresh horehound leaves per cup of hot water. Steep for 10 minutes. Strain and sip ½ cup three times a day, for no more than two consecutive weeks. Sweeten to taste. Make fresh daily.

PROPERTIES: appetite stimulant, carminative, diaphoretic, diuretic, expectorant, stimulant, tonic

This perennial plant is native to Europe, the Mediterranean, and Asia, and has been an effective expectorant for thousands of years. Horehound is found in over-the-counter cough and throat medicines.

WARNING: DO NOT TAKE INTERNALLY WHILE PREGNANT. MAY CAUSE MISCARRIAGE.

HORSETAIL *(Equisetum spp.)*

SPANISH: *cola de caballo*

THERAPEUTIC USES: anemia, arthritis, chest infection, kidney disorders

PARTS USED: whole plant

APPLICATION:

POULTICE: Crush and chop ½ to 1 cup fresh or dried horsetail stems. Add enough hot water or oil to act as a binder. Dab olive oil on skin, then apply the poultice to the affected area. Cover with gauze or a towel. Make fresh daily.

TEA/INFUSION: 1 teaspoon dry or 2 teaspoons fresh horsetail stems per cup of hot water. Steep for 10 minutes. Strain and sip ½ cup three times a day, for no more than two consecutive weeks. Sweeten to taste. Make fresh daily.

PROPERTIES: anti-inflammatory, antispasmodic, astringent, diuretic, hemostatic, vulnerary

WARNING: DO NOT EXCEED PRESCRIBED DOSAGE. DO NOT TAKE IF YOU HAVE HYPERTENSIVE DISEASE OR CARDIOVASCULAR PROBLEMS. DO NOT REPLACE HORSETAIL WITH MARSH HORSETAIL (*EQUISETUM PALUSTRE*). THE LATTER IS HIGHLY TOXIC.

Horsetail is indigenous to Asia, Africa, and Europe, and has been around since the Paleozoic era (600–375 million years ago). Though this perennial looks like a horse's tail, it is poisonous to livestock. Horsetail is rich in silica, which accounts for its ability to restore tissue. Horsetail's diuretic uses are universal. It also contains vitamin B, nicotine, thiamin, riboflavin, and niacin, along with ascorbic acid.

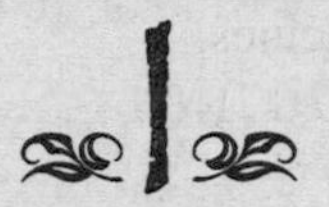

INDIAN PAINTBRUSH (*Castileja spp.*)

SPANISH: *flor de Santa Rita*

THERAPEUTIC USES: contraception, water retention

PARTS USED: flowers, leaves

APPLICATION:

DECOCTION: In a saucepan add 1 teaspoon dried or 3 teaspoons chopped fresh Indian paintbrush leaves per cup of cold water. Cover and simmer for 15 minutes. Strain and sip ½ cup of the decoction three times a day. Sweeten to taste. Make fresh daily.

PROPERTIES: anti-inflammatory, diuretic

This perennial is indigenous to South America, where it has long been used as a diuretic and at one time as a treatment for leprosy. It is often plucked by children for its honey.

INDIAN ROOT (*Aristolochia spp.*)

SPANISH: *yerba del indio, raíz del indio*

THERAPEUTIC USES: flu, stomachache, toothache, vaginal infection

PARTS USED: root, leaves

DECOCTION: In a saucepan add 1 teaspoon dried and crushed or 2 teaspoons chopped fresh Indian root per cup of cold water. Cover and simmer for 30 minutes or until liquid is reduced by ⅓. Strain and sip ½ cup of the decoction three times a day, for no more than two weeks. Add honey to taste. Make fresh daily.

POULTICE: Crush and chop ½ to 1 cup fresh or dried Indian root. Add enough hot water or oil to act as a binder. Dab olive oil on skin before applying the poultice to the affected area. Cover with gauze or a towel. Make fresh daily.

TINCTURE: Add 1 part Indian root to 3 parts alcohol (at least 80 proof) and 2 parts water. Store in a dark, cool place for a week or two. (Never use rubbing alcohol [isopropyl alcohol]; it is extremely toxic if taken internally.) Strain liquid into an airtight glass container. Take 20 drops in a glass of juice or water, two or three times a day. Two-year shelf life.

PROPERTIES: antibacterial, antiseptic, stomachic

WARNING: DO NOT TAKE INTERNALLY WHILE PREGNANT OR BREASTFEEDING. DO NOT USE WHILE TAKING PRESCRIPTION MEDICINE. DO NOT EXCEED PRESCRIBED DOSAGE.

Indigenous to Europe, the genus name of this perennial, *Aristolochia*, means "expedient birth." This is due to its early uses for inducing labor. Some species contain alkaloid acids, which invigorate white blood cells but may also act as a carcinogen.

INDIAN TOBACCO *(Nicotiana rustica)*

SPANISH: *punche Mexicano*

THERAPEUTIC USES: arthritis, asthma, broken bones, chest cold, cramps, earache, headache, rheumatism

PART USED: leaves

APPLICATION:

OIL: Heat ½ cup olive oil in a double boiler. Add 3 tablespoons crushed Indian tobacco leaves, then heat for an additional 20 minutes. Strain warm liquid into an airtight glass container. One-year shelf life.

OINTMENT/SALVE: Slowly heat ⅓ to ½ cup lard or petroleum jelly in a double boiler over low heat. Add 2 or 3 tablespoons finely chopped Indian tobacco leaves and heat for an additional 30 minutes. Strain and store in an airtight glass container. Two-year shelf life.

POULTICE: Crush and chop ½ to 1 cup fresh or dried Indian tobacco leaves. Add enough hot water or oil to act as a binder. Dab olive oil on skin before applying the poultice to the affected area. Cover with gauze or a towel. Make fresh daily.

PROPERTIES: anodyne, narcotic

WARNING: INDIAN TOBACCO CONTAINS LARGE DOSES OF NICOTINE AND IS CLASSIFIED AS A NARCOTIC.

This annual and biennial plant is indigenous to Central America. The Maya were familiar with the medicinal uses of tobacco, treating asthma and skin conditions with the leaves. Indian tobacco contains alkaloids, such as nicotine, and volatile oils, which absorb quickly into the skin.

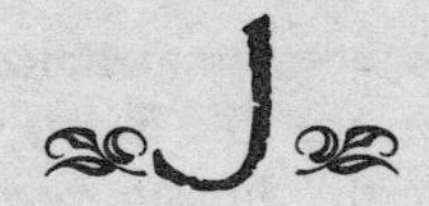

JALAPEÑO

SPANISH: *jalapeño*

THERAPEUTIC USE: insect bites

These pungent little green peppers are an outstanding source of vitamin A.

JIMSON WEED *(Datura stramonium)*

SPANISH: *toloache*

THERAPEUTIC USES: abscesses, aches, arthritis, asthma, boils, headache, hemorrhoids, rattlesnake bite, sprains, swelling, tumors

PARTS USED: flowers, leaves, seeds

APPLICATION:

INFUSION: 1 teaspoon dry or 2 teaspoons fresh jimson weed per cup of hot water. Steep for 10 minutes. Do not take internally. Make fresh daily.

OINTMENT/SALVE: Slowly heat ⅓ to ½ cup lard or petroleum jelly in a double boiler over low heat. Add 2 or 3 tablespoons finely chopped jimson weed, then heat for an additional hour. Strain and store in an airtight glass container. Two-year shelf life.

POULTICE: Crush and chop ½ to 1 cup fresh or dried jimson weed. Add enough hot water or oil to act as a binder. Dab olive oil on skin, then apply the poultice to the affected area. Cover with gauze or a towel. Make fresh daily.

PROPERTIES: anodyne, antibiotic, antispasmodic, narcotic

WARNING: FOR EXTERNAL USE ONLY, POISONOUS IF TAKEN INTERNALLY.

Jimson weed has been immortalized on canvases by Georgia O'Keeffe. In the Old West, this annual was referred to as "loco weed." Jimson weed can be traced back to the Aztecs for much of the same uses. It contains tropane alkaloids, which are poisonous if taken internally.

JUNIPER (*Juniperus spp.*)

SPANISH: *sabino, sabina*

THERAPEUTIC USES: appetite stimulant, menstrual flow

PARTS USED: berries, needles

APPLICATION:

DECOCTION: In a saucepan add 1 teaspoon dried and crushed or 2 teaspoons fresh juniper needles per cup of cold water. Cover and simmer for 30 minutes or until liquid is reduced by ⅓. Add to a warm bath.

PROPERTIES: antiseptic, carminative, diuretic, rubefacient, stomachic

WARNING: DO NOT TAKE INTERNALLY WHILE PREGNANT OR WHILE BREASTFEEDING; MAY CAUSE MISCARRIAGE. DO NOT USE IF YOU HAVE KIDNEY DISORDERS. DO NOT EXCEED PRESCRIBED DOSAGE.

Most people are familiar with the flavor that juniper berries lend to gin and other liqueurs. The juniper berry was a common laxative used by the ancient Egyptians. Recent research indicates that although the oil from the berries is an effective diuretic, it may irritate the kidneys. The essential oil is an active ingredient in over-the-counter diuretics.

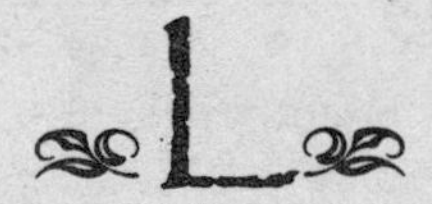

LARD

SPANISH: *manteca*

THERAPEUTIC USES: abscesses, aches, arthritis, burns, fever

Lard is made from pork fat that has been melted, clarified, then cooled. It is widely used in Mexican cooking and in folk medicine. Traditionally, lard is cleaned by placing it in a shallow vessel then mixing and rinsing saltwater and vinegar through it several times. The final rinse takes alcohol. Prepared lard is also available in the United States.

LAUREL/BAY (*Laurus nobilis*)

SPANISH: *laurel*

THERAPEUTIC USES: appetite stimulant, colds, headache, insect repellent

PART USED: leaves

APPLICATION:

STEAM INHALATION: In a pot or old teakettle, simmer a

strong infusion or decoction of bruised and chopped laurel over low heat. Remove from heat source. Drape a towel over your head and inhale the steam.

TEA/INFUSION: 1 teaspoon dry or 2 teaspoons chopped fresh laurel leaves per cup of hot water. Steep for 10 minutes. Strain and sip ½ cup three times a day. Sweeten to taste. Make fresh daily.

PROPERTIES: appetite stimulant, astringent, carminative, digestive, stomachic, tonic.

This evergreen shrub is indigenous to the Mediterranean region. The genus name, *Laurus*, derives from *laus*, which is Latin for "praise," referring to the crown of laurel worn by the conquering Romans. Laurel leaves are still worn under hats throughout the Southwest, though they are now believed to act as an insect repellent.

LAVENDER (*Lavandula spp.*)

SPANISH: *alhucema*

THERAPEUTIC USES: asthma, colic, coughs, cramps, disinfectant, flatulence, fumigation, indigestion, lactation, miscarriage, stomachache

PARTS USED: flowers, leaves

APPLICATION:

POULTICE: Crush and chop ½ to 1 cup fresh or dried lavender flowers. Add enough hot water or oil to act as a binder. Dab olive oil on skin, then apply the poultice to the affected area. Cover with gauze or a towel. Make fresh daily.

TEA/INFUSION: 1 teaspoon dry or 2 teaspoons fresh lavender flowers and leaves per cup of hot water. Steep for 10 minutes. Strain and sip ½ cup three times a day. Sweeten to taste. Make fresh daily.

PROPERTIES: antibacterial, antidepressant, antiseptic, antispasmodic, carminative, cholagogue, diuretic, febrifuge, sedative, stomachic

Native to the Mediterranean region and France, lavender's name derives from the Latin word *lavare*, "to wash." The ancient Phoenicians and Egyptians were the first to bottle this fragrant herb. The efficacy of lavender is due in part to the volatile oil in the flowers.

LEMON (*Citrus limon*)

SPANISH: *limón*

THERAPEUTIC USES: cancer, calcium deficiency, colds, cuts, fever, gas, hangover, hiccups, insect bites, nerves, scars, sinus infection, sore throat, sty, *susto*, varicose veins

PARTS USED: leaves, fruit, flowers, peel, seeds

APPLICATION:

STEAM INHALATION: In a pot or old teakettle, simmer a strong infusion or decoction of lemon over low heat. Remove from heat source. Drape a towel over your head and inhale the steam.

TEA/INFUSION: 1 teaspoon dry or 2 teaspoons fresh leaves, peels and/or flowers per cup of hot water. Steep for 10 minutes. Strain and sip 1 cup three times a day. Sweeten to taste. Make fresh daily.

PROPERTIES: antibacterial, anti-inflammatory, antiseptic, febrifuge, tonic

Indigenous to Asia, this evergreen is a popular folk remedy on both sides of the Atlantic. Italy and southern California supply just about the entire world with lemons. Lemons are interchangeable with limes in Mexico. Both are an important preventive agent, and are a rich source of vitamins A, B_1, and C; acids; coumarins; and volatile oil. They are also high in potassium.

LEMONGRASS (*Cymbopogon citratus*)

SPANISH: *té de limón*

THERAPEUTIC USES: fever, stomachache, stress

PARTS USED: leaves
APPLICATION:
TEA/INFUSION: 1 teaspoon dry or 2 teaspoons fresh lemongrass leaves per cup of hot water. Steep for 10 minutes. Strain and sip ½ cup three times a day. Make fresh daily.
PROPERTIES: analgesic, antibacterial

Though indigenous to India, this perennial is now grown in most temperate regions. Lemongrass contains citral, which can also be found in lemon peels. This grass contains volatile oil, which is an effective sedative.

LIME (*Citrus aurantifolia*)

SPANISH: *lima*
THERAPEUTIC USES: colds, hiccups, insect bites, liver disorders
PARTS USED: leaves, fruit, flowers, peel, seeds
APPLICATION:
TEA/INFUSION: 1 teaspoon dry or 2 teaspoons fresh lime leaves per cup of hot water. Steep for 10 minutes. Strain and sip ½ cup three times a day. Make fresh daily.
PROPERTIES: antibacterial, antiseptic, ferbifuge

In Mexico, a distinction is not always made between lemons and limes. Mexican American folk remedies have given each fruit its own therapeutic properties. Limes are rich in vitamin C and B_1 and contain potassium.

LINDEN (*Tilia spp.*)

SPANISH: *tila*
THERAPEUTIC USES: cramps, depression, insomnia, *susto*
PARTS USED: flowers, leaves
APPLICATION:
TEA/INFUSION: 1 teaspoon dry or 2 teaspoons fresh flowers or leaves per cup of hot water. Steep for 10

minutes. Strain and sip ½ cup three times a day. Make fresh daily.

PROPERTIES: antispasmodic, diaphoretic, diuretic, sedative, stomachic

The relaxing effects of this deciduous tree have been known since the Middle Ages. Sitting under the tree was believed to be a cure for epilepsy.

LIZARD TAIL (*Anemopsis californica*)

SPANISH: *yerba mansa*

THERAPEUTIC USES: arthritis, bruises, colds, colic, diaper rash, gums, hemhorroids, menstrual cramps, scrapes, sinus infections, stomachache, ulcers, vaginal infection

PARTS USED: leaves, root

APPLICATION:

DECOCTION: In a saucepan add 1 teaspoon dried and crushed or 3 teaspoons chopped fresh lizard tail root per cup of cold water. Cover and simmer for 30 minutes or until liquid is reduced by ⅓. Strain and sip ½ cup of the decoction three times a day. Add honey to taste. Make fresh daily.

POULTICE: Crush and chop ½ to 1 cup fresh or dried lizard tail plant. Add enough hot water or oil to act as a binder. Dab olive oil on skin before applying the poultice to the affected area. Cover with gauze or a towel. Make fresh daily.

TEA/INFUSION: 1 teaspoon dry or 2 teaspoons fresh lizard tail leaves per cup of hot water. Steep for10 minutes. Strain and sip ½ cup four times a day. Make fresh daily.

TINCTURE: Add 1 part lizard tail root to 3 parts alcohol (at least 80 proof) and 2 parts water. (Never use rubbing alcohol [isopropyl alcohol]; it is extremely toxic if taken internally.) Store in a dark, cool place for a week or two. Strain liquid into an airtight glass container. Two-year shelf life.

PROPERTIES: analgesic, antibacterial, antifungal, anti-inflammatory, antiseptic, sedative

This native plant is one of the most respected medicinal herbs in the southwestern United States and Mexico. Its name means "tamed Indian."

LOVAGE (*Ligusticum porteri*)

SPANISH: *oshá, chuchupate*

THERAPEUTIC USES: *aire*, asthma, *bilis*, broken bones, chest colds, coughs, cramps, cuts, fever, hangover, rattlesnake bite, stomachache, toothache, witchcraft

PART USED: root

APPLICATION:

DECOCTION: In a saucepan add 1 teaspoon dried and crushed or 3 teaspoons chopped fresh lovage root per cup of cold water. Cover and simmer for 30 minutes or until liquid is reduced by ⅓. Strain and sip ½ cup of the decoction three times a day. Sweeten to taste. Make fresh daily.

POULTICE: Crush and chop ½ to 1 cup fresh or dried lovage root. Add enough hot water or oil to act as a binder. Dab olive oil on skin, then apply the poultice to the affected area. Cover with gauze or a towel. Make fresh daily.

TEA/INFUSION: 1 teaspoon dry or 2 teaspoons grated fresh lovage root per cup of hot water. Steep for 10 minutes. Strain and sip ½ cup three times a day, for no more than two consecutive weeks. Sweeten to taste. Make fresh daily.

TINCTURE: Add 1 part bruised lovage root to 3 parts alcohol (at least 80 proof) and 2 parts water. (Never use rubbing alcohol [isopropyl alcohol]; it is extremely toxic if taken internally.) Store in a dark, cool place for a week or two. Strain liquid into an airtight glass container. Take 30 drops in a glass of juice or water, two or three times a day. Two-year shelf life.

PROPERTIES: anti-inflammatory, carminative, diuretic, emmenagogue, expectorant, stimulant, stomachic

This perennial is reputed to be effective for anything from snakebites to seasoning food. Lovage contains volatile and fixed oils, and a very bitter alkaloid that has been shown to increase blood flow to the coronary arteries and the brain.

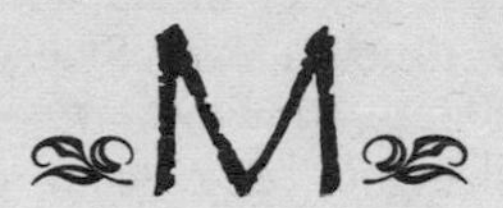

MAIDENHAIR FERN (*Adiantum spp.*)

SPANISH: *culantrillo*

THERAPEUTIC USES: coughs, hair, menstrual stimulant

PARTS USED: leaves, root

APPLICATION:

DECOCTION: In a saucepan add 1 teaspoon dried and crushed or 2 teaspoons chopped fresh maidenhair fern root per 2 cups of cold water. Cover and simmer for 15 minutes. Strain and sip when thirsty. Add honey to taste. Make fresh daily.

TEA/INFUSION: 1 tablespoon dry or 2 tablespoons fresh maidenhair leaves per cup of hot water. Steep for 10 minutes. Strain and sip 2 cups a day. Sweeten to taste. Make fresh daily.

PROPERTIES: antispasmodic, expectorant, tonic

WARNING: DO NOT TAKE INTERNALLY WHILE PREGNANT OR WHILE BREASTFEEDING.

This feathery perennial plant is indigenous to the tropical regions of South America, where it has been used for coughs and as a hair rinse since ancient times. Plant derivatives are found in over-the-counter cough medicines.

MALLOW *(Malva spp.)*

SPANISH: *malva*

THERAPEUTIC USES: afterbirth, diaper rash, pimples, stomachache, vaginal infection

PART USED: whole plant

APPLICATION:

COLD DECOCTION: Steep 1 teaspoon dried and crushed or 3 teaspoons of chopped fresh mallow plant per cup of cold water, overnight. Strain and sip ½ cup of the decoction three times a day. Sweeten to taste. Make fresh daily.

PROPERTIES: astringent, demulcent, emmenagogue, expectorant, mucilage

Mallow has been in use as a medicine for over a thousand years. The ancient Aztecs utilized this plant for childbirth.

MARIJUANA *(Cannabis sativa)*

SPANISH: *marijuana*

THERAPEUTIC USE: bone cancer, rheumatism

PARTS USED: leaves, stems

APPLICATION:

POULTICE: Crush and chop ½ to 1 cup fresh or dried marijuana leaves and stems. Add enough hot water or oil to act as a binder. Dab olive oil on skin, then apply the poultice to the affected area. Cover with gauze or a towel. Make fresh daily.

TINCTURE: Add 1 part marijuana leaves and stems to 5 parts alcohol (at least 80 proof). Store in a dark, cool place for a week or two. Strain liquid into an airtight glass container. Do not take internally. Two-year shelf life.

PROPERTIES: anti-inflammatory, hallucinogenic

WARNING: ILLEGAL IN THE UNITED STATES.

Native to the Caucasus, Northern India, and Iran, marijuana has been in medicinal and religious use for the past 5,000 years. Its narcotic properties were recognized close to 3,000 years ago in Asia. Marijuana has been utilized by royalty such as Queen Victoria, who employed the herb as an analgesic.

MATÉ (*Ilex paraguayensis*)

SPANISH: *yerba maté*
THERAPEUTIC USE: appetite suppressant, hangover
PART USED: leaves
APPLICATION:
TEA/INFUSION: 1 teaspoon dry or 2 teaspoons fresh maté leaves per cup of hot water. Steep for 10 minutes. Strain and sip ½ cup three times a day. Sweeten to taste. Make fresh daily.
PROPERTIES: diuretic, stimulant

WARNING: DO NOT EXCEED PRESCRIBED DOSAGE. DO NOT TAKE INTERNALLY IF YOU ARE AVOIDING CAFFEINE.

The dried leaves of this holly bush have been drunk as a tea in South America for centuries. The primary ingredient is caffeine (2 percent).

MESQUITE (*Prosopis juliflora*)

SPANISH: *mesquite*
THERAPEUTIC USES: diarrhea, *empacho*, eye irritation
PARTS USED: sap, bark, leaves, pods
APPLICATION:
DECOCTION: In a saucepan add 1 teaspoon dried and crushed or 3 teaspoons chopped fresh mesquite per cup of cold water. Cover and simmer for 30 minutes or until liquid is reduced by ⅓. Strain and sip ½ cup of the

decoction three times a day. Sweeten to taste. Make fresh daily.

EYE WASH: Boil 2 cups of water and add ¼ teaspoon salt and 1 teaspoon crushed mesquite pod. Let cool, then strain and use. Make fresh daily.

PROPERTIES: antibacterial, astringent

Native to the Southwest, this tree is commonly used as a medicine. The bean pods are a food source in the southwestern and northern Mexico, containing 805 total carbohydrates. Mesquite is also a good source of protein and fiber.

MINT (*Mentha spicata/M. piperita*)

SPANISH: *yerba buena, hierba buena*

THERAPEUTIC USES: aches, colds, cramps, digestion, *empacho*, hangover, headache, labor, lactation, morning sickness, nausea, stomachache

PARTS USED: leaves, stems

APPLICATION:

OINTMENT/SALVE: Slowly heat ⅓ cup to ½ cup lard or petroleum jelly in a double boiler over low heat. Add 2 or 3 tablespoons finely chopped mint leaves, then heat for an additional hour. Strain and store in an airtight glass container. Two-year shelf life.

TEA/INFUSION: 1 teaspoon dry or 2 teaspoons fresh mint leaves per cup of hot water. Steep for 10 minutes. Strain and sip ½ cup three times a day. Make fresh daily.

TINCTURE: Add 1 part mint to 5 parts alcohol (at least 80 proof). (Never use rubbing alcohol [isopropyl alcohol]; it is extremely toxic if taken internally.) Store in a dark, cool place for a week or two. Strain liquid into an airtight glass container. Take 20 drops in a glass of juice or water, two or three times a day. Two-year shelf life.

PROPERTIES: antiseptic, carminative, diaphoretic, stimulant, stomachic

Peppermint has no known origins since it appears to be a hybrid of spearmint and water mint. Thus, spearmint and peppermint are often interchanged in Mexico. Mint is both refreshing and tepid to the senses. With over 600 species, mint is still continuing to hybridize.

MORMON TEA *(Ephedra trlfurcu)*

SPANISH: *cañutillo, tepopote*

THERAPEUTIC USES: asthma, hay fever, kidney stones, stomachache

PARTS USED: twigs, leaves

APPLICATION:

TEA/INFUSION: 1 teaspoon dry or 2 teaspoons fresh Mormon tea per cup of hot water. Steep for 10 minutes. Strain and cool. Sip ½ cup three times a day, for no more than two consecutive weeks. Sweeten to taste. Make fresh daily.

PROPERTIES: antispasmodic, diuretic, febrifuge, stimulant, tonic

WARNING: TAKE UNDER A PHYSICIAN'S SUPERVISION. MORMON TEA RAISES BLOOD PRESSURE.

The Mormon settlers, who had refrained from drinking coffee or tea, were accepting of this beverage. This tea was popular long before the Aztec reign. In fact, vestiges of this herb were discovered in a Neolithic site that goes back 60,000 years.

MOUNTAIN BALM *(Eriodictyon californicum)*

SPANISH: *yerba santa*

THERAPEUTIC USES: asthma, bronchitis, colds, coughs, hay fever, neck stiffness, sinus infection, sore throat

PART USED: leaves

APPLICATION:

POULTICE: Crush and chop ½ to 1 cup fresh or dried mountain balm. Add enough hot water or oil to act as a binder. Dab olive oil on skin before applying the poultice to the affected area. Cover with gauze or a towel. Make fresh daily.

TEA/INFUSION: 1 teaspoon dry or 2 teaspoons fresh mountain balm per cup of hot water. Steep for 10 minutes. Strain and sip ½ cup three times a day, for no more than two consecutive weeks. Sweeten to taste. Make fresh daily.

PROPERTIES: antispasmodic, disinfectant, expectorant, febrifuge

This evergreen shrub is native to the western United States and is widely known for its expectorant properties. The name *yerba santa* is Spanish for "holy weed." Native Americans inhaled the smoke from the dry leaves to relieve asthma. They also chewed on the leaves to relieve colds and to freshen breath. Today, mountain balm can be found in cough medicines as an expectorant and to mask the flavor of the medicine.

MUIRA-PUAMA (*Liriosma ovata*)

SPANISH: *raíz del Macho*

THERAPEUTIC USES: aphrodisiac, impotence, sore throat

PARTS USED: bark, root

APPLICATION:

DECOCTION: In a saucepan add 1 teaspoon dried and crushed or 3 teaspoons freshly chopped muira-puama root per cup of cold water. Cover and simmer for 30 minutes or until liquid is reduced by ⅓. Strain and sip ½ cup of the decoction three times a day. Add honey to taste. Make fresh daily.

PROPERTIES: astringent, stimulant

WARNING: DO NOT TAKE INTERNALLY WHILE PREGNANT OR BREASTFEEDING. DO NOT TAKE DURING MENSTRUAL CYCLE. DO NOT EXCEED PRESCRIBED DOSAGE.

For centuries, this shrub has been used as a powerful aphrodisiac in South American folk medicine. Preliminary research indicates that muira-puama is safe and effective, improving libido and sexual function in some patients.

MULLEIN (*Verbascum thapsus*)

SPANISH: *gordolobo, punchón*

THERAPEUTIC USES: asthma, bronchitis, coughs, fever, gallstones, hemorrhoids, respiratory problems, spider bites

PARTS USED: leaves, flowers

APPLICATION:

POULTICE: Crush and chop ½ to 1 cup fresh or dried mullein leaves and flowers. Add enough hot water or oil to act as a binder. Dab olive oil on skin, then apply the poultice to the affected area. Cover with gauze or a towel. Make fresh daily.

TEA/INFUSION: 1 teaspoon dry or 2 teaspoons fresh mullein leaves and flowers per cup of hot water. Steep for 10 minutes. Strain and sip ½ cup three times a day. Sweeten to taste. Make fresh daily.

TINCTURE: Add 1 part bruised leaves to 5 parts alcohol (at least 80 proof). (Never use rubbing alcohol [isopropyl alcohol]; it is extremely toxic if taken internally.) Store in a dark cool place for a week or two. Strain liquid into an airtight container. Take 20 to 30 drops in a glass of juice or water, two or three times a day. Two-year shelf life.

PROPERTIES: anodyne, antiseptic, antispasmodic, demulcent, diuretic, expectorant, vulnerary

Since early times, this biennial has been used to cure physical ailments and get rid of evil spirits. Mullein contains a high quantity of mucilage and has a slightly bitter taste.

MUSTARD (*Brassica nigra/B. hirta*)

SPANISH: *mostaza*

THERAPEUTIC USE: aches, fever

PARTS USED: black and white seeds

APPLICATION:

POULTICE: Pulverize ½ to 1 cup mustard seeds. Add enough cold water to act as a binder. Apply the poultice to the soles of the feet. Cover with gauze or a towel. If mustard plaster is too hot upon contact, add water. Make fresh daily.

PROPERTIES: appetite stimulant, digestive, rubefacient

WARNING: IF IRRITATION DEVELOPS, RINSE OFF SKIN IMMEDIATELY AND DISCONTINUE USE.

The ingredients in table mustard have not changed much since Roman times. There are several types of mustard seed: black, brown, white, and oriental. Though all are effective in poultices, the black seeds tend to have more of a bite.

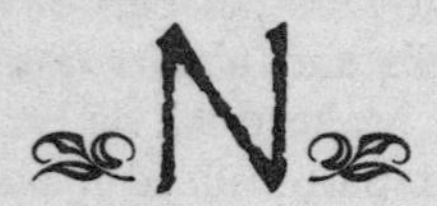

NUTMEG *(Myristica fragrans)*

SPANISH: *nuez moscada*

THERAPEUTIC USES: flatulence, hangover, stomachache

PART USED: seeds

APPLICATION:

DECOCTION: In a saucepan add 1 teaspoon dried and crushed nutmeg per cup of cold water. Cover and simmer for 30 minutes or until liquid is reduced by ⅓. Strain and sip ½ cup of the decoction three times a day. Sweeten to taste. Make fresh daily.

PROPERTIES: carminative, hallucinogenic

WARNING: DO NOT EXCEED PRESCRIBED DOSAGE; NUTMEG CAN BE HIGHLY TOXIC AND HALLUCINOGENIC.

This evergreen tree is native to Indonesia and was once believed to be an aphrodisiac. Nutmeg and mace are cultivated from the same fruit; nutmeg is the seed, and mace is the fruity growth that envelops it. Though they are similar in taste, nutmeg tends to be a bit on the bitter side.

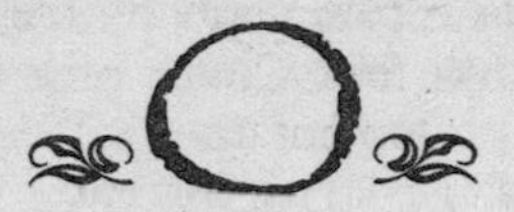

Oak (*Quercus gambelii*)

Spanish: *encino*

Therapeutic uses: fever, skin cancer, water retention

Parts used: leaves, bark

Application:

cold infusion: Add 1 teaspoon dried or 3 teaspoons chopped fresh bark and leaves per cup of cold water. Let sit overnight. Strain and drink. Make fresh daily.

decoction: In a saucepan add 1 teaspoon dried and crushed or 3 teaspoons chopped fresh bark and leaves per cup of cold water. Cover and simmer for 30 minutes or until liquid is reduced by ⅓. Strain and sip ½ cup of the decoction three times a day. Sweeten to taste. Make fresh daily.

Properties: astringent, diuretic, ferbifuge

The oak tree was very popular during biblical times. Abraham was visited by God near an oak tree (Genesis 13: 18 and 18:1). Ancient Europeans believed that the mighty oak tree could never be struck by lightning. Over a hundred species of this deciduous and evergreen tree grow in Mexico.

Onion (*Allium cepa*)

Spanish: *cebolla*

Therapeutic uses: burns, coughs, cramps, earache, flatulence, labor, lung conditions, respiratory problems, scalds

Part used: bulb

Application:

COMPRESS: Soak a clean cloth made of cotton in a hot or cold infusion, decoction, or tincture.

POULTICE: Crush and chop ½ to 1 cup fresh onions. Dab olive oil on skin before applying the poultice to the affected area. Cover with gauze or a towel. Make fresh daily.

PROPERTIES: analgesic, antibiotic, anti-inflammatory, antiseptic, aphrodisiac, diuretic, expectorant, stimulant, stomachic, vermifuge

Onions are part of almost every culture's folk medicine and lore. This perennial plant is part of the lily family. The sulfur compounds found in onions act as an antiseptic and are helpful to the liver. The same antiseptic is also effective for all types of respiratory infections and as an expectorant for coughs. When ingested, raw onions may lower cholesterol and blood pressure, and aid in circulation and digestion. Onions contain vitamins A, C, and D; thiamine; and riboflavin.

ORANGE, SEVILLE *(Citrus aurantium)*

SPANISH: *naranja*

THERAPEUTIC USE: burns, cramps, hangover, nerves

PARTS USED: fruit, rind, leaves, blossoms

APPLICATION:

TEA/INFUSION: 1 teaspoon dry or 2 teaspoons fresh orange rind and blossom per cup of hot water. Steep for 10 minutes. Strain and sip ½ cup three times a day. Make fresh daily.

PROPERTIES: antibacterial, anti-inflammatory, antispasmodic, carminative, febrifuge, stomachic, tonic

Native to Asia, the fruit from this evergreen tree has been cultivated since ancient times. The citrus family is made up of eighteen species, including lemons, limes, and tangerines. The blossoms contain neroli oil, a stimulant said to act as an aphrodisiac. Oranges also contain bergamot oil, which is said to have sedative and healing properties.

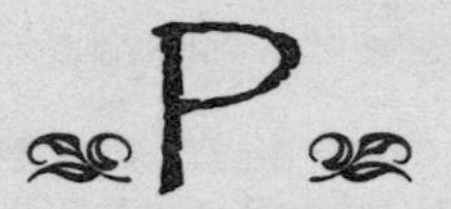

PAPAYA (*Carica papaya*)

SPANISH: *papaya*

THERAPEUTIC USES: indigestion, jellyfish stings, wounds

PARTS USED: fruit, leaves

APPLICATION:

POULTICE: Crush and chop ½ to 1 cup fresh papaya leaves. Add enough hot water or oil to act as a binder. Dab olive oil on skin before applying the poultice to the affected area. Cover with gauze or a towel. Make fresh daily.

PROPERTIES: digestive, stomachic, vermifuge, vulnerary

This herbaceous tree is indigenous to Central America. The pulpy fruit has long been used by the various Indian groups of Mexico in the treatment of cuts and wounds. Papaya leaves are used to tenderize meat. Papain, the enzyme in this tropical fruit, can consume 35 times its own weight in protein foods. Papaya is rich in vitamins A, C, and E, and contains phosphorus, calcium, and iron.

PARSLEY (*Petroselinum sativum*)

SPANISH: *perejil*

THERAPEUTIC USES: blood pressure, cramps, gums, headaches, nosebleeds

PARTS USED: whole plant, seeds

APPLICATION:

POULTICE: Crush and chop ½ to 1 cup fresh parsley. Add enough hot water or oil to act as a binder. Dab olive oil on skin before applying the poultice to the affected area. Cover with gauze or a towel. Make fresh daily.

TEA/INFUSION: 1 teaspoon dry or 2 teaspoons fresh parsley leaves per cup of hot water. Steep for 10 minutes. Strain and sip ½ cup three times a day. Make fresh daily.

PROPERTIES: antispasmodic, carminative, diuretic, emmenagogue, expectorant, hemostatic, nervine, tonic

WARNING: DO NOT EXCEED INTERNAL DOSAGE WHILE PREGNANT OR BREASTFEEDING.

This annual or biennial plant is native to the Mediterranean region. The Greeks adorned the tombs of their loved ones with parsley; it was symbolic of a new beginning. Parsley is a rich source of iron, and contains copper, calcium, potassium, phosphorus, sulfer, and vitamins A, C, and E.

PASSIONFLOWER *(Passiflora incarnata)*

SPANISH: *pasionaria*
THERAPEUTIC USE: bruises, insomnia
PARTS USED: flowers, leaves
APPLICATION:

POULTICE: Crush and chop ½ to 1 cup fresh or dried passionflower. Add enough hot water or oil to act as a binder. Dab olive oil on skin before applying the poultice to the affected area. Cover with gauze or a towel. Make fresh daily.

TEA/INFUSION: 1 teaspoon dry or 2 teaspoons fresh passionflowers and leaves per cup of hot water. Steep for 10 minutes. Strain and sip ½ cup three times a day. Sweeten to taste. Make fresh daily.

TINCTURE: Add 1 part plant to 5 parts alcohol (at least 80 proof). (Never use rubbing alcohol [isopropyl alcohol]; it is extremely toxic if taken internally.) Store in a dark cool place for a week or two. Strain liquid into an airtight container. Take 20 to 40 drops in a glass of juice or water, two or three times a day. Two-year shelf life.

PROPERTIES: antispasmodic, sedative

WARNING: DO NOT TAKE INTERNALLY WHILE PREGNANT OR BREASTFEEDING, OR IF SUFFERING FROM KIDNEY DISORDERS.

When the Spaniards first came upon this vine, they dubbed it ''passion flower.'' Since they were so far from home, we can only speculate that this was a way to pay homage to the crucifixion of Jesus Christ. The Spaniards noticed many symbolic parallels between Christ and this distinctive flower. They noted a crown of thorns and the nails in the three stigmata, the wounds were the five stamens; and the ten sepals were representative of the ten apostles (Judas Iscariot had betrayed the Lord, and Peter had denied him). Indigenous to the southern regions of the United States and Central, and South America, over 400 species have been counted. Native Americans have long since used the leaves of this perennial for bruises. Passionflower contains nonaddictive sedatives.

PEYOTE *(lophophora williamsii)*

SPANISH: *Peyote*

THERAPEUTIC USES: arthritis, fever, headaches, rheumatism

PART USED: whole plant

APPLICATION:

TINCTURE: Add 1 part peyote to 5 parts alcohol (at least 80 proof). Store in a dark, cool place for a week or two. Strain liquid into an airtight glass container. For external use only. Two-year shelf life.

PROPERTIES: antibiotic, cardiac, stimulant, hallucinogenic, narcotic

WARNING: ILLEGAL IN THE UNITED STATES. HIGHLY HALLUCINOGENIC.

This spineless cactus is native to Mexico and Texas. Historically, peyote or *peyotl* was used in the ceremonial practices of northern Mexico's high priests. Mescaline buttons were consumed by the Indians, who would then experience what they perceived to be an intense spiritual encounter. Though it is considered to be a psychedelic, peyote is actually akin to amphetamines. Peyote contains the hallucinogen mescaline, which in measured doses invigorates the heart and respiratory system.

PINE (*Pinus spp.*)

SPANISH: *piñon*

THERAPEUTIC USES: burns, energy, joints, scars, splinters, water retention

PARTS USED: bark, oil, needles

APPLICATION:

OINTMENT: Heat pine pitch and lard. Once mixture turns into a liquid, remove from heat, strain, and apply. The ointment will keep for several months.

TEA/INFUSION: 1 teaspoon dry or 2 teaspoons fresh pine needles per cup of hot water. Steep for 10 minutes. Strain and sip 3 cups a day. Add honey to taste. Make fresh daily.

TINCTURE: Add 1 part pine needles to 3 parts alcohol (at least 80 proof) and 2 parts water. (Never use rubbing alcohol [isopropyl alcohol]; it is extremely toxic if taken internally.) Store in a dark, cool place for a week or two. Strain liquid into an airtight container. Two-year shelf life.

PROPERTIES: antiseptic, diuretic, stimulant

WARNING: IF A RASH OCCURS, RINSE OFF SKIN AND DISCONTINUE USE

There are close to 100 species of this evergreen tree growing in most continents. Pine's medical history goes back to ancient times, when turpentine was first tapped.

PLANTAIN (*Plantago major*)

SPANISH: *llantén*

THERAPEUTIC USES: abcesses, athlete's foot, boils, constipation, headache, insect bites, poison ivy, swelling, tumors

PARTS USED: flower spikes, leaves

APPLICATION:

POULTICE: Crush and chop ½ to 1 cup fresh or dried plantain leaves. Add enough hot water or oil to act as a binder. Dab olive oil on skin before applying the poultice to the affected area. Cover with gauze or a towel. Make fresh daily.

TEA/INFUSION: 1 teaspoon dry or 2 teaspoons fresh plantain leaves per cup of hot water. Steep for 10 minutes. Strain and sip ½ cup three times a day. Make fresh daily.

PROPERTIES: anti-inflammatory, astringent, decongestant, demulcent, diuretic, expectorant, hemostatic

Not to be mistaken with the species of cooking banana with the same name, this plantain was dubbed by Native Americans as "white man's foot," due to its spreading throughout the continents by way of the explorers. The seeds were dropped from the tangled hides of the livestock, and supposedly from the cuffs of the trailblazers' pants, onto the soil of the new frontier.

POTATO *(Solanum tuberosum)*

SPANISH: *papa*

THERAPEUTIC USES: eye inflammation, fevers, headache, insect bites, mumps, sunburn

PART USED: tuber

APPLICATION:

POULTICE: ½ to 1 cup freshly grated potatoes. Add enough hot water or oil to act as a binder. Dab olive oil on skin before applying the poultice to the affected area. Cover with gauze or a towel. Make fresh daily.

PROPERTIES: astringent, febrifuge, stomachic

This versatile vegetable is actually native to Bolivia, Chile, and Peru. Sir Francis Drake is said to have introduced this vegetable to England and Ireland in the sixteenth century. Over 1,500 species are included in the *Solanum* genus. Potatoes are a rich source of vitamin C, and also contain vitamins A, B, and K. This perennial also contains potassium and starch. Though the tubers are edible, the leaves contain toxic alkaloids.

PRICKLY-PEAR CACTUS/BEAVERTAIL CACTUS (*Opuntia spp.*)

SPANISH: *nopal*

THERAPEUTIC USES: diabetes, diarrhea, sunburn, water retention

PARTS USED: fruit, pads

APPLICATION:

POULTICE: Crush and chop ½ to 1 cup peeled and mashed cactus. Add enough hot water or oil to act as a binder. Dab olive oil on skin before applying the poultice to the affected area. Cover with gauze or a towel. Make fresh daily.

PROPERTIES: anti-inflammatory, diuretic, hypoglycemic

This perennial cactus is indeginous to Mexico. In ancient times, Aztecs used the plant for skin conditions. Prickly-pear cactus has been proven to be effective in reducing blood sugar levels.

PRUNE (*Prunus domestica*)

SPANISH: *ciruela*

THERAPEUTIC USE: colds

PART USED: fruit

PROPERTIES: laxative, lubricant, stomachic

WARNING: DO NOT EXCEED DOSAGE. EXCESSIVE QUANTITIES OF PRUNES MAY PRODUCE CRAMPS AND STOMACHACHE.

Native to Western Asia, plums were cultivated by the Spanish priests at the Mission Santa Clara in California as early as 1792. Most people are familiar with the laxative efficacy of dried plums or prunes, which contain dietary fiber.

PUMPKIN (*Curcurbita pepo*)

SPANISH: *calabaza*

THERAPEUTIC USES: headache, tapeworms

PARTS USED: pulp, seed
APPLICATION:
DECOCTION: In a saucepan add 1 teaspoon dried and crushed pumpkin seeds per cup of cold water. Cover and simmer for 30 minutes or until liquid is reduced by ⅓. Strain and sip ½ cup of the decoction three times a day. Sweeten to taste. Make fresh daily.
POULTICE: Crush and chop ½ to 1 cup fresh pumpkin pulp. Apply the poultice onto the affected area. Cover with gauze or a towel. Make fresh daily.
PROPERTY: anthelmintic

This annual is indigenous to both America and Europe. The Maya made an ointment for burns from the pulp and sap. The fruit is rich in potassium and sodium and also contains zinc. Pumpkin is also a good source for beta carotene and fiber. The seeds contain various minerals and vitamins.

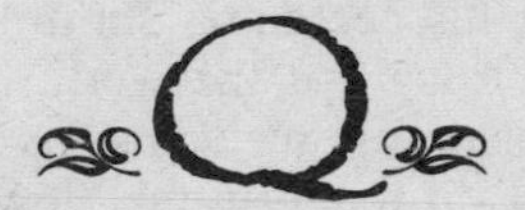

QUASSIA (*Picrasma excelsum*)

SPANISH: *cuasia*
THERAPEUTIC USES: appetite stimulant, *coraje*, digestion
PARTS USED: bark, wood
APPLICATION:
COLD DECOCTION: Steep 1 teaspoon quassia shavings per cup of cold water, then let sit out overnight. Strain and sip ½ cup of the decoction three times a day. Sweeten to taste. Make fresh daily
PROPERTIES: stomachic, tonic

WARNING: DO NOT EXCEED PRESCRIBED DOSAGE. MAY CAUSE VOMITING.

This deciduous tree is indigenous to tropical America and the West Indies. A bitter resin can be extracted from the wood. Quassia contains vitamin B.

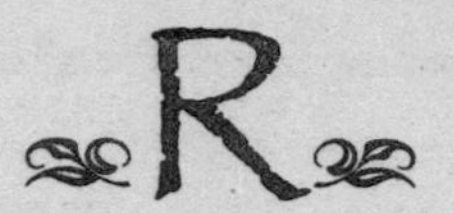

Rose *(Rosa spp.)*

Spanish: *rosa de Castilla*

Therapeutic uses: colic, constipation, diaper rash, earache, eye irritation, fever, skin care, sore throat, stomachache, vaginal infection

Parts used: flowers, hips

Application:

eye wash: Boil 1 cup water, and add ¼ teaspoon salt or 1 teaspoon rose petals. Let cool, then strain and use. Make fresh daily.

tea/infusion: 1 teaspoon dry or 2 teaspoons fresh rose petals per cup of hot water. Steep for 10 minutes. Strain and sip ½ cup three times a day. Sweeten to taste. Make fresh daily.

Properties: antibacterial, astringent, stomachic

Native to Iran, this deciduous shrub has over 100 species and blooms throughout the world. The red rose has been part of European folk medicine for centuries. Attar of rose is an essential oil found in this flower that acts as an antidepressant. The fruits, or rosehips, are a rich source of vitamin C, and also contain vitamins A, B, and K.

Rosemary *(Rosmarinus officinalis)*

Spanish: *romero*

Therapeutic uses: *aire*, colds, contraception, digestion, disinfectant, *empacho, espanto*, menstrual stimulant, skin care, *susto*, vaginal infection

Parts used: leaves, flowers

Application:

tea/infusion: 1 teaspoon dry or 2 teaspoons fresh rosemary per cup of hot water. Steep for 10 minutes. Strain and sip ½ cup three times a day, for no more than two consecutive weeks. Sweeten to taste. Make fresh daily.

tincture: Add 1 part rosemary to 5 parts alcohol (at

least 80 proof). (Never use rubbing alcohol [isopropyl alcohol]; it is extremely toxic if taken internally.) Store in a dark, cool place for a week or two. Strain liquid into an airtight glass container. Take 20 drops in a glass of juice or water, two or three times a day. Two-year shelf life.

PROPERTIES: anti-inflammatory, astringent, carminative, emmenagogue, nervine, stimulant, stomachic, tonic

WARNING: DO NOT EXCEED INTERNAL DOSAGE WHILE PREGNANT OR WHILE BREAST-FEEDING.

This evergreen shrub is indigenous to the Mediterranean region. Rosemary was worn to improve memory by the ancient Greeks, and was the symbol of love and fidelity. Hardy and aromatic, this plant has been considered a panacea for female ailments for centuries. In Mexico, a rosemary infusion is used to help bring on one's period and ease the pain of cramps, and a douche is commonly utilized by prostitutes as a form of birth control. As a preventive of scars in the ritual of self-mortification, whips are first dipped in an infusion of rosemary. Rosemary contains phenolic acids, which are a strong antiseptic.

RUE *(Ruta graveolens)*

SPANISH: *ruda*

THERAPEUTIC USES: *aire*, colic, diaper rash, earache, headache, menstrual stimulant

PART USED: leaves

APPLICATION:

OIL: Heat ½ cup olive oil in a double boiler. Add 3 tablespoons crushed rue, then heat for an additional 20 minutes. Strain warm liquid into an airtight glass container. One-year shelf life.

TEA/INFUSION: 1 teaspoon dry or 2 teaspoons fresh rue leaves per cup of hot water. Steep for 10 minutes. Strain and sip ½ cup three times a day. Make fresh daily.

TINCTURE: Add 1 part rue to 5 parts alcohol (at least 80

proof). (Never use rubbing alcohol [isopropyl alcohol]; it is extremely toxic if taken internally.) Store in a dark, cool place for a week or two. Strain liquid into an airtight glass container. Take 15 to 30 drops in a glass of juice or water, two or three times a day. Two-year shelf life.

PROPERTIES: antispasmodic, carminative, emmenagogue, stimulant, stomachic

WARNING: DO NOT TAKE INTERNALLY WHILE PREGNANT; RUE MAY CAUSE MISCARRIAGE. DO NOT TAKE WHILE BREASTFEEDING OR IF YOU HAVE A LIVER DISORDER. DISCONTINUE EXTERNAL USE IF RASH DEVELOPS.

This evergreen perennial is native to the Mediterranean. In the past, priests in the Catholic church would dip branches of rue in holy water, then sprinkle the parishioners during Mass. Both Michelangelo and Leonardo da Vinci reported rue to be effective for enhancing their ability to create art. A derivative of rue is can be found in some commercial ear medications.

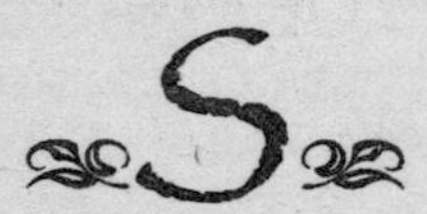

SAFFLOWER/MEXICAN SAFFRON

(Carthamus tinctorius)

SPANISH: *azafrán*

THERAPEUTIC USES: fever, measles

PART USED: flowers

APPLICATION:

TEA/INFUSION: 1 teaspoon dry or 2 teaspoons fresh safflower per cup of hot water. Steep for 10 minutes. Strain and sip ½ cup three times a day. Sweeten to taste. Make fresh daily.

PROPERTIES: anti-inflammatory, ferbifuge

WARNING: DO NOT TAKE FLOWERS INTERNALLY WHILE PREGNANT OR BREASTFEEDING.

This annual plant is indigenous to the Mediterranean region, and has been discovered in ancient Egyptian tombs. Safflower extract is yellow when added to water, but turns red in alcohol. It is used as a dye for food and clothing. In the eighteenth century, saffron was a scarce delicacy in Portugal, and safflower or "false saffron" was used in its place.

SAGE (*Salvia officinalis*)

SPANISH: *salvia*

THERAPEUTIC USES: diabetes, gums, infertility, insomnia, nerves, weaning

PART USED: leaves

APPLICATION:

TEA/INFUSION: 1 teaspoon dry or 2 teaspoons fresh sage per cup of hot water. Steep for 10 minutes. Strain and sip ½ cup three times a day, for no more than two consecutive weeks. Sweeten to taste. Make fresh daily.

TINCTURE: Add 1 part sage to 5 parts alcohol (at least 80 proof). (Never use rubbing alcohol [isopropyl alcohol]; it is extremely toxic if taken internally.) Store in a dark cool place for a week or two. Strain liquid into an airtight glass container. Take 30 drops in a glass of juice or water, two or three times a day. Two-year shelf life.

PROPERTIES: antispasmodic, astringent, carminative, tonic

WARNING: DO NOT TAKE INTERNALLY WHILE PREGNANT OR BREASTFEEDING.

With over 900 species, this perennial plant has been in continuous use for thousands of years. Its popularity peaked in the Middle Ages when sage elixirs were bottled and sold throughout Europe. Salvia is Latin for "health" or "to heal." Sage tea is still a popular tea in Greece.

SALT *(sodium chloride)*

SPANISH: *sal*

THERAPEUTIC USE: *caida de la mollera*, eye wash, headache, insect bite, sore throat

Salt has a well-rounded history. Its uses include currency, ritual practices, and food preparation and preservation. In Latin *sal* means "wit." In Spanish, *sal* is also a colloquialism for inciting bad luck or a curse on another person. *Salar* or "to salt" means to place a curse on an individual.

SARSAPARILLA, MEXICAN *(Smilax aristolochiaefolia)*

SPANISH: *zarzaparrillà, mecapatili*

THERAPEUTIC USES: aphrodisiac, blood tonic, hives, tuberculosis

PART USED: root

APPLICATION:

DECOCTION: In a saucepan add 1 teaspoon dried or 3 teaspoons fresh sarsaparilla root per cup of cold water. Cover and simmer for 30 minutes or until liquid is reduced by ⅓. Strain and sip ½ cup of the decoction three times a day. Sweeten to taste. Make fresh daily.

PROPERTIES: carminative, diaphoretic, diuretic, tonic

This perennial is native to Australia and Asia, and has long been used in Mexico as an aphrodisiac.

SASSAFRAS *(Sassafras officinale)*

SPANISH: *sasafrás*

THERAPEUTIC USE: blood tonic

PART USED: bark

APPLICATION:

DECOCTION: In a saucepan add 1 teaspoon dried or 3 teaspoons chopped fresh sassafras bark per cup of cold water. Cover and simmer for 30 minutes or until liquid is reduced by ⅓. Strain and sip ½ cup of the decoction three times a day. Sweeten to taste. Make fresh daily.

PROPERTIES: antiseptic, diaphoretic, diuretic, stimulant

WARNING: DO NOT EXCEED PRESCRIBED DOSAGE. DO NOT TAKE INTERNALLY WHILE PREGNANT. MAY CAUSE MISCARRIAGE. DO NOT TAKE INTERNALLY WHILE BREASTFEEDING.

It is said that sassafras is the first plant introduced to Europe from America. The volatile oil consists of 80 to 90 percent safrole and acts as a mucus membrane irritant.

SENNA *(Cassia Spp.)*

SPANISH: *sena*

THERAPEUTIC USE: constipation

PART USED: leaves

APPLICATION:

DECOCTION: In a saucepan add 1 teaspoon dried and crushed or 3 teaspoons chopped fresh senna leaves per cup of cold water. Cover and simmer for 30 minutes or until liquid is reduced by ⅓. Strain and sip ½ cup of the decoction three times a day. Sweeten to taste. Make fresh daily.

PROPERTIES: cathartic, diuretic, stimulant, vermifuge

WARNING: DO NOT EXCEED PRESCRIBED DOSAGE. NOT RECOMMENDED FOR CHILDREN OR SENIOR CITIZENS. MAY CAUSE CRAMPING AND ABDOMINAL PAIN.

Indigenous to northern Africa and North America, senna was being utilized as a laxative by the Aztecs prior to the arrival of the Spaniards. Senna contains sennosides, an extract from senna leaves found in many over-the-counter laxatives.

STAR ANISE (*Illicium spp.*)

SPANISH: *anís de estrella*

THERAPEUTIC USES: appetite stimulant, colic, flatulence, insomnia

PART USED: seeds

APPLICATION:

TEA/INFUSION: 1 teaspoon dry seeds per cup of hot water. Steep for 10 minutes. Strain and sip ½ cup three times a day. Sweeten to taste. Make fresh daily.

TINCTURE: Add 1 part star anise seeds to 3 parts alcohol (at least 80 proof) and 2 parts water. (Never use rubbing alcohol [isopropyl alcohol]; it is extremely toxic if taken internally.) Store in a dark, cool place for a week or two. Strain liquid into an airtight glass container. Take 10 to 20 drops in a glass of juice or water. Two-year shelf life.

PROPERTIES: antibacterial, carminative, stimulant, stomachic

This evergreen tree is native to China and Vietnam. Star anise is similar to fennel and aniseed, yet is of no relation. Star anise contains the volatile oil anethole, a mild stimulant.

STONECROP (*Sedum spp.*)

SPANISH: *siempreviva*

THERAPEUTIC USES: backache, corns, cramps, dysentery, earache, headache, scalds, stomachache

PART USED: leaves

APPLICATION:

POULTICE: Crush and chop ½ to 1 cup fresh or dried stonecrop. Add enough hot water or oil to act as a binder. Dab olive oil on skin before applying the poultice to the affected area. Cover with gauze or a towel. Make fresh daily.

TEA/INFUSION: 1 teaspoon dry or 2 teaspoons fresh st[...] crop leaves per cup of hot water. Steep for 10 minutes. Strain and sip ½ cup three times a day, for no more than two consecutive weeks. Sweeten to taste. Make fresh daily.

Stonecrop is a succulent, often transplanted by *yerberas* to their gardens for their practices.

SUNFLOWER (*Helianthus annuus*)

SPANISH: *girasol*
THERAPEUTIC USES: arthritis, nerves, rheumatism
PART USED: whole plant
APPLICATION:
TEA/INFUSION: 1 teaspoon dry or 2 teaspoons fresh sunflower per cup of hot water. Steep for 10 minutes. Strain and sip ½ cup three times a day. Make fresh daily.

Indigenous to the Americas, this emblem of the sun has been part of Indian medicine and lore for over 3,000 years. Each flower head produces around 1,000 seeds, which contain vitamin E. Sunflowers also contain yellow dye and fixed oil.

SWEET CLOVER/MELILOT (*Melilotus officinalis*)

SPANISH: *alfalfón.*
THERAPEUTIC USES: air freshener, breasts, headache, moth repellent
PARTS USED: flowers, leaves
APPLICATION:
POULTICE: Crush and chop ½ to 1 cup fresh or dried sweet clover. Add enough hot water or oil to act as a binder. Dab olive oil on skin before applying the poultice to the affected area. Cover with gauze or a towel. Make fresh daily.
PROPERTIES: antispasmodic, aromatic

This biennial plant is native to Europe and North Africa, but has been naturalized in North America. Sweet clover has the scent of freshly mown hay, and is cultivated as fodder. Fermented sweet clover is used for rat poison. Sweet clover contains coumarin, which gives it a vanilla aroma.

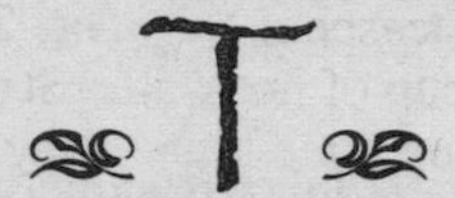

THYME *(Thymus spp.)*

SPANISH: *tomillo*

THERAPEUTIC USES: asthma, bronchitis, fumigation, headache, sore throat

PART USED: leaves

APPLICATION:

TEA/INFUSION: 1 teaspoon dry or 2 teaspoons fresh thyme leaves per cup of hot water. Steep for 10 minutes. Strain and sip ½ cup three times a day, for no more than two consecutive weeks. Sweeten to taste. Make fresh daily.

TINCTURE: Add 1 part thyme to 3 parts alcohol (at least 80 proof), and two parts water. (Never use rubbing alcohol [isopropyl alcohol]; it is extremely toxic if taken internally.) Store in a dark, cool place for a week or two. Strain liquid into an airtight glass container. Take 20 drops in a glass of juice or water, two or three times a day. Two-year shelf life.

PROPERTIES: anti-inflammatory, antiseptic, antispasmodic, carminative, diaphoretic, expectorant, sedative, tonic.

Thyme has been of medicinal use for coughs and lung disorders since antiquity. The Greeks made incense from thyme, hence its name, *thyein*, "to smoke." Thyme contains the volatile oil thymol, which relieves asthma by relaxing the bronchial tubes, and it is an effective antiseptic.

TRUMPET BUSH (*Tecoma stans*)

SPANISH: *tronadora, trompetilla, palo de Arco, flor de San Pedro*

THERAPEUTIC USES: diabetes, liver disorders

PARTS USED: branches, flowers

APPLICATION:

TEA/INFUSION: 1 teaspoon dry or 2 teaspoons fresh trumpet bush per cup of hot water. Steep for 10 minutes. Strain and sip ½ cup three times a day. Make fresh daily.

PROPERTIES: antibiotic, antidiabetic, anti-inflammatory

WARNING: CONSULT YOUR PHYSICIAN BEFORE TAKING FOR DIABETES.

This shrub, native to southern New Mexico, Arizona, and northern Mexico, is a common remedy for diabetes. This herb is excellent for the treatment of insulin resistant diabetes. Trumpet flower contains acids which act as a liver stimulant.

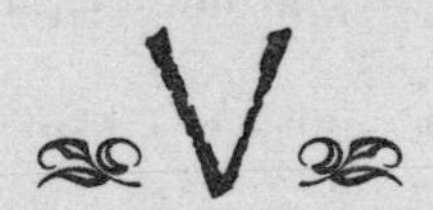

VALERIAN (*Valeriana officinalis*)

SPANISH: *valeriana*

THERAPEUTIC USES: insomnia, nerves, stomachache

PARTS USED: leaves, rhizomes, root

APPLICATION:

DECOCTION: In a saucepan add 1 teaspoon dried and crushed or 3 teaspoons chopped fresh valerian plant per cup of cold water. Cover and simmer for 30 minutes or until liquid is reduced by ⅓. Strain and sip ½ cup of the decoction three times a day. Sweeten to taste. Make fresh daily.

TINCTURE: Add 1 part valerian plant to 3 parts alcohol (at least 80 proof) and 2 parts water. (Never use rubbing alcohol [isopropyl alcohol]; it is extremely toxic if taken internally.) Store in a dark, cool place for a week or two. Strain liquid into an airtight glass container. Take 30 drops as needed. Two-year shelf life.

PROPERTIES: antispasmodic, calmative, carminative, stomachic

WARNING: MAY CAUSE DROWSINESS. DO NOT TAKE WHILE PREGNANT OR BREAST-FEEDING.

This perennial plant is native to Europe and northern Asia. As a mild tranquilizer, valerian has been used for close to 2,000 years. Valerian is often confused with Valium, a trademark used for diazepam. Valerian contains valeporiats, which produce sedative effects.

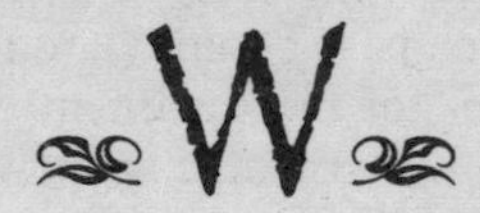

WILD GOURD (*Cucurbita foetidissima)*

SPANISH: *calabazilla.*

THERAPEUTIC USES: insect repellent, laundry soap, shampoo

PARTS USED: fruit, pulp, seeds

APPLICATION:

DECOCTION: In a saucepan add 1 pounded and chopped wild gourd to 1 liter cold water. Cover and simmer for 1 hour or until liquid is reduced by ⅓. Strain and bottle.

This plant has been used as a wash by Native Americans for centuries. A lather is created by the saponins contained within the gourd.

WILLOW (*Salix spp.)*

SPANISH: *jarita, saúz*

THERAPEUTIC USES: arthritis, bladder infections, fever, headache

PARTS USED: bark, leaves

APPLICATION:

DECOCTION: In a saucepan add 1 teaspoon dried and crushed willow bark per cup of cold water. Cover and simmer for 30 minutes or until liquid is reduced by ⅓. Strain and sip ½ cup of the decoction twice a day. Sweeten to taste. Make fresh daily.

PROPERTIES: analgesic, anti-inflammatory, antiseptic, astringent, diuretic, febrifuge, tonic

WARNING: DO NOT TAKE IF YOU ARE ALLERGIC TO ASPIRIN.

Native to Europe, this deciduous tree has been used for baskets, tanning materials, and reducing fevers for over 2,000 years. The bark and leaves of willow contain salicylic acid, a relation to acetylsalicylic, the basis for aspirin.

WORMSEED/MEXICAN TEA *(Chenopodium ambrosioides)*

SPANISH: *epazote, pazote*

THERAPEUTIC USES: *aire*, *espanto*, lactation, menstrual cramps, menstrual stimulant, postpartum care, stomachache, worms

PARTS USED: leaves, seeds

APPLICATION:

DECOCTION: In a saucepan add 1 teaspoon dried and crushed wormseed per cup of cold milk. Cover and simmer for 10 minutes or until liquid is reduced by ⅓. Strain and sip ½ cup of the decoction three times a day. Sweeten to taste. Make fresh daily.

TEA/INFUSION: 1 teaspoon dry or 2 teaspoons fresh wormseed per cup of hot water. Steep for 10 minutes. Strain and sip ½ cup twice a day. Sweeten to taste. Make fresh daily.

PROPERTIES: anthelmintic, antispasmodic, emmenagogue, galactogogue

WARNING: DO NOT ADMINISTER OIL TO SMALL CHILDREN. DO NOT USE WHILE PREGNANT. DO NOT EXCEED PRESCRIBED DOSAGE. WORMSEED IS TOXIC IN LARGE DOSES.

Indigenous to Central America, wormseed contains ascaridol, which, as Native Americans have known for centuries, gives the plant the ability to expel worms. This annual is a popular seasoning in Mexican kitchens, and is often added to the flavoring of beans and corn.

WORMWOOD *(Artemisia ludoviciana)*

SPANISH: *estafiate, ajenjo*

THERAPEUTIC USES: *bilis*, diarrhea, *empacho*, headache, stomachache

PARTS USED: flowers, leaves

APPLICATION:

TEA/INFUSION: 1 teaspoon dry or 2 teaspoons fresh wormwood per cup of hot water. Steep for 10 minutes. Strain and sip ½ cup three times a day, for no more than one week. Sweeten to taste. Make fresh daily.

TINCTURE: Add 1 part wormwood to 3 parts alcohol (at least 80 proof) and 2 parts water. (Never use rubbing alcohol [isopropyl alcohol]; it is extremely toxic if taken internally.) Store in a dark, cool place for a week or two. Strain liquid into an airtight container. Take 20 drops in a glass of juice or water, two or three times a day, for no more than two days. Two-year shelf life.

PROPERTIES: anti-inflammatory, antiseptic, antispasmodic, carminative, cholagogue, febrifuge, stomachic

WARNING: DO NOT USE INTERNALLY WHILE PREGNANT OR BREASTFEEDING. DO NOT EXCEED PRESCRIBED DOSAGE. MAY BE TOXIC. DO NOT TAKE WITH PRESCRIPTION

MEDICINE. PROFESSIONAL SUPERVISION IS RECOMMENDED.

Vincent van Gogh cut off his ear while under the influence of absinthe, a French aperitif whose primary ingredient is wormwood. The genus name *Artemisia* originated with Artemis, the Greek goddess of women, hence its longstanding association with female medicinals. Absinthe has been banned in most countries, including France. This perennial plant is considered a panacea among Mexicans and Chicanos. Wormwood was used for rituals by the Aztecs as well as for physical ailments. It contains the volatile oil abithol and highly toxic thujone, which may be toxic if taken excessively.

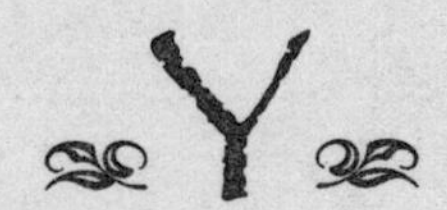

YARROW (*Achillea millefolium*)

SPANISH: *plumajillo*

THERAPEUTIC USES: colds, fever, insect repellent, menstrual flow, stomachache, ulcers, wounds

MEDICINAL PARTS USE: flower tops, leaves

APPLICATION:

POULTICE: Crush and chop ½ to 1 cup fresh or dried yarrow plant. Add enough hot water or oil to act as a binder. Dab olive oil on skin before applying the poultice to the affected area. Cover with gauze or a towel. Make fresh daily.

TEA/INFUSION: 1 teaspoon dry or 2 teaspoons fresh yarrow per cup of hot water. Steep for 10 minutes. Strain and sip ½ cup three times a day. Make fresh daily.

PROPERTIES: anti-inflammatory, antiseptic, antispasmodic, astringent, diaphoretic, febrifuge, hemostatic

WARNING: DO NOT TAKE INTERNALLY WHILE PREGNANT OR BREASTFEEDING. IF CONTACT DERMATITIS OCCURS, DISCONTINUE USE.

This feathery perennial plant has quite a military history. *Achillea*, the genus name of the plant, refers to the Greek warrior Achilles. Native American warriors treated wounds with the leaves, as did World War I infantrymen. The species name, *millefolium*, means "thousand-leaved." Yarrow is a potent medicine with over 50 distinctive constituents. They include rutin and quercetin, which is similar to aspirin.

YUCCA (*Yucca spp.*)

SPANISH: *amole*
USES: shampoo, soap
PART USED: root
APPLICATION:

DECOCTION: In a saucepan add equal parts chopped yucca root and cold water. Cover and simmer until liquid becomes thick. Strain into an airtight glass container.

WARNING: DISCONTINUE USE IF SKIN BECOMES IRRITATED.

The joshua tree (*Y. brevifolia*), a member of this species, grows in the United States and Mexico.

Chapter 5

The Sources

The following is a list of retail and wholesale herbal companies. Consult your local phone directory or health-food store for retailers in your neighborhood.

Alive and Wild Herbals
P.O. Box 5654,
Bisbee, AZ 85603-5654
(520) 432-7679

Southwestern bulk herbs, tinctures and oils. Wholesale and retail.

Central Naturista de Baja California
857 Ridgewater Dr.
Chula Vista, CA 91913

Herbs grown in Mexico.

El Milagro Herbs
P.O. Box 123
Gila, NM 88038
(505) 535-4135

Specialty orders. Unique formulations. *Se habla español.*

The Herb Shoppe
Box 395
Duenweg, MO 64841
(417) 782-0457
E-mail:herbshoppe@
talleytech.com

Specializing in medicinal combinations.

Horizon Herbs

P.O. Box 69
Williams, OR 97544
(541) 846-6704
E-mail:
herbseed@chatlink.com

Free catalog/growing guide. Three hundred types of medicinal seeds.

Moonrise Herbs

826 G Street
Arcata, CA 95521
(800) 603-8364

Mail-order catalog available.

Southwestern Native Seeds

P.O. Box 50503
Tucson, AZ 85703

Seeds native to the southwestern United States and Mexico.

Sage Woman Herbs, Ltd.

2211 W. Colorado Ave.
Colorado Springs, CO
80904
(719) 473-9702
http://www.funtimes.com/
sagewoman.html

Herbs in bulk, tinctures, oils, and so on.

Wildseed Inc.

1101 Campo Rosa Rd,
P.O. Box 308
Eagle Lake,Texas 77434
Phone: (409) 234-7353,
Fax: (409) 234-7407

Informative catalog $1.00.

Web Sites and Links of Interest

Algy's Herb Page
http://www.algy.com/herb

Arizona Cactus & Succulent Research, Inc.
http://www.arizonacactus.com

Internet Directory for Botany
http://www.helsinki.fi/kmus/whatsnew.html

Joe and Mindy's Herbal Links
http://www.nhn.uoknor.edu/~howard/herbs.html

Medicinas Tradicionales y Alternativas
http://www.cam.org/%7Etlahuic/medici.htm

Places to Find Herbal Remedies
http://www.kohala.net/health/herbs.html

Poisonous Plant Database
http://www.inform.umd.edu/PBIO/Medicinals/harmful.html

The Ethnobotany Cafe
http://countrylife.net/ethnobotany

National Organizations

American Botanical Council
P.O. Box 201660
Austin, TX 78720
(512) 331-8868
http://www.herbalgram.org

Herb Research Foundation
1007 Pearl St., Suite 200
Boulder, CO 80302
(303) 449-2265
http:/www.herbs.org

American Herbalists Guild
Box 1683
Soquel, CA 95073
(408) 464-2441
http://www.healthy.net/herbalists/

Glossary

Alkaloid: A nitrogen-containing compound, occurring in plants and some fungi, that has poisonous or medicinal attributes.

Analgesic: A substance that reduces pain at a conscious level.

Anesthetic: An agent that blocks nerve impulses from the affected part without loss of vital function.

Annual: A plant that completes its life cycle in one year or growing season.

Anodyne: A substance that abates pain.

Anthelmintic: An agent that expels parasitic worms.

Antibacterial: A substance that eradicates or inhibits the growth of bacteria.

Antibiotic: An agent that destroys or inhibits the growth and spreading of microorganisms.

Antifungal: An agent that acts against fungal infections.

Anti-inflammatory: An agent that reduces swelling.

Antipyretic: A substance that reduces or prevents fever.

Antiseptic: A substance that prevents the growth of microorganisms that cause infection.

Antispasmodic: An agent that relieves or reduces muscle spasm.

Aperient: A gentle laxative.

Aphrodisiac: A drug that excites the sexual functions.

Appetizer: An agent that increases the appetite.

Aromatic: A plant with high levels of volatile oil producing a pleasant odor and stimulating qualities.

Astringent: 1) A pore cleanser. 2) A substance that shrinks the tissue.

Atole: Corn gruel.

Barrida: A cleansing ritual in which a person is spiritually swept to alleviate emotional, physical, or spiritual problems.

Biennial: A plant that flowers and dies every two years after germination.

Bilis: The belief that some stomach illnesses are caused by lingering anger and fear.

Bitter: A substance that stimulates secretion of saliva and digestive juices, which improves appetite.

Bruise: To crush the membrane of a plant.

Calmative: A substance that contains a mild sedative.

Carcinogen: A cancer-causing substance.

Carminative: A substance used to relieve colic, griping, and flatulence.

Cathartic: An extreme laxative or purgative.

Cholagogue: An agent that promotes the movement of bile through the intestines.

Colic: Stomach pains that cause strong contractions of the intestines or bladder.

Compress: A cloth soaked in a hot or cold liquid and applied to the skin.

Coumarin: A vanilla-scented plant constituent.

Crudo: Hangover.

Curandera/curandero: A folk healer of Mexican origin, whose ability to heal derives from "white magic."

Deciduous: A plant that sheds its leaves annually.

Decoction: A method of extracting medicinals from plants or bark with boiling water.

Decongestant: An agent that alleviates congestion in the nasal passages.

Demulcent: A medicinal liquid that lubricates and protects the tissue.

Diaphoretic: An agent that increases perspiration, lowering fever.

Disinfectant: A substance used to destroy bacteria that cause disease.

Diuretic: An agent that stimulates urinary flow.

Don, el: "The gift" to heal.

Dysentery: Inflammation of the large intestine accompanied by diarrhea.

Emmenagogue: Any agent that stimulates menstrual flow.

Emollient: A softening agent applied externally.

Empacho: A condition caused by food that is lodged in the intestines and will not pass.

Enema: A liquid injection into the rectum used to evacuate the bowels.

Espanto: Fright or loss of soul.

Essence: 1) Fragrance. 2) A solution of alcohol, water, and plant extract.

Essential oil: A volatile oil derived from a plant, distinctive of the plant.

Expectorant: An agent that promotes coughing and helps discharge phlegm from the throat and chest.

Extract: A concentration of a solution.

Febrifuge: A substance that reduces or removes fever.

Fixed oil: A nonvolatile oil.

Galactogogue: An agent that increases milk flow.

Hallucinogenic: An agent that induces visions or hallucinations.

Hemostatic: An agent that serves to stop or reduce bleeding.

Herbaceous: A plant that dies down at the end of the growing season.

Homeopathy: Minute doses of a substance that would in a healthy person create the same symptoms as in the diseased person being treated.

Humor: Body fluid.

Hypoglycemia: A deficiency of blood glucose.

Infusion: Expulsion of the vital ingredients through soaking in water.

Inhalation: Consumption of medicine by means of inhaling.

Lactation: Production of milk by the mammary glands, which usually begins at the end of pregnancy.

Laxative: A substance used in the relief of constipation.

Lubricant: Application of oil on skin to reduce swelling.

Materia Medica: Resources used to prepare remedies.

Medicinal: A curative used in the treatment of disease.

Mucilage: A viscous carbohydrate secreted by certain plants.

Narcotic: A drug that induces mental lethargy, reduces pain, and can produce sleep.

Nervine: An agent that soothes the nerves. Also called *nerve tonic.*

Ointment: Oil or cream that forms a protective layer over the skin.

Ojo de venado: Buckeye seed carried to deflect the evil eye.

Partera: Midwife.

Perennial: A plant that continues to live from year to year without replanting.

Plantilla: A poultice for the feet.

Poultice: A heated herbal preparation spread on a cloth and administered to sore or inflamed areas.

Purgative: A substance that causes strong evacuation of the intestines.

Remedios caseros: Home remedies.

Rhizome: A branched underground storage stem.

Rubefacient: An agent that stimulates blood flow to skin, which increases the blood flow and cleansing of toxins.

Saline: A substance containing common salt.

Salve: A curative or soothing ointment.

Sanalotodo: Cure-all, panacea.

Saponins: A group of soaplike glycosides, found widely in plants, that have complex effects in herbal remedies; some resemble steroidal hormones.

Sedative: A calming, tranquilizing agent that abates the nervous system.

Sereno: A preparation of tea left out at night.

Sobador/sobadora: massage therapist.

Stimulant: A substance that provides a temporary increase in functional activity.

Stomachic: An agent that eases stomach pain and strengthens stomach activity.

Succulent: A plant with thick, lush leaves and/or stems.

Sudorific: A sweat-inducing agent.

Susto: Fright or loss of soul.

Syrup: A concentration of sugar and liquid.

Tannin: An agent which contracts tissue.

Terpenes: Complex organic macromolecules that form the base of most constituents of volatile oils.

Thymol: A element in volatile oil that acts as an antiseptic, fungicide, and vermifuge.

Tincture: A liquid consisting of a medicinal substance and alcohol.

Tonic: A substance that restores the body by stimulating the tissue.

Tuber: A thickened underground storage organ.

Vermifuge: An agent that expels intestinal worms.

Volatile oil: A plant constituent distilled to procure essential oil.

Vulnerary: An agent that heals wounds.

Yerbera/yerbero: A person whose field of expertise is with herbs and herbal remedies.

***Yerberia*:** An herb store; synonymous with *botica.*

Bibliography

Arias-Carvajal, Pio. *Plantas que Curan y Plantas que Matan: Tratado Teórico Practico de Botanica Medicinal para la Curación de Todas las Enfermedades.* Mexico, Ediciones Ciceron, 1952.

Ballesteros, Octavio A., Ed.d. *Mexican Proverbs: The Philosophy, Wisdom and Humor of a People.* Burnet, TX: Eakin Press, 1979.

Beidermann, Hans. *Dictionary of Symbolism: Cultural Icons and the Meanings Behind Them.* New York: Meridian, 1994.

Bremness, Lesley. *The Complete Book of Herbs.* New York: Viking Studio Books, 1994.

Brown, Deni. *Encyclopedia of Herbs & Their Uses.* New York: Dorling Kindersley, Limited, 1995.

Burciaga, Jose Antonio. *In Few Words: En Pocas Palabras: A Compendium of Latino Folk Wit and Wisdom.* San Francisco: Mercury House, 1997.

Carrasco, Sara M. Campos. *Mexican-American Folk Medicine: A Descriptive Study of the Different Curanderismo Techniques Practiced by Curanderos or Curanderas and Used by Patients in the Laredo, Texas Area* (Dissertation) 1984.

Castleman, Michael. *The Healing Herbs: The Ultimate Guide to the Curative Power of Nature's Medicines.* Emmaus, PA: Rodale Press, 1991.

Chevallier, Andrew. *The Encyclopedia of Medicinal Plants.* New York: Dorling Kindersley Publishing Inc., 1996.

Chiej, Roberto. *The Macdonald Encyclopedia of Medicinal Plants.* London: Macdonald & Co., Ltd. 1984.

Coon, Nelson. *Using Plants for Healing.* Emmaus, PA: Rodale Press, 1979.

de Waal, Marinus, Ph.D. *Medicines From the Bible: Roots & Herbs & Woods & Oils.* York Beach, ME: Samuel Weiser, Inc., 1994.

Duke, James A. *Medicinal Plants of the Bible.* New York: Trado-Medic Books, 1983.

Emmart, Emily Walcott. *The Badianus Manuscipt.* Baltimore, MD: John Hopkins University Press. 1940.

Etkin, Nina L. *Plants in Indigenous Medicine & Diet: Biobehavioral Approaches.* Bedford Hills, NY: Redgrave Publishing Company, 1986.

Folk Wisdom of Mexico (Proverbios y Dichos Mexicanos). San Francisco: Chronicle Books, 1994.

Ford, Karen Cowan. *Las Yerbas de la Gente: A Study of Hispano-American Medicinal Plants.* Ann Arbor, MI: University of Michigan, 1975.

Harris, Ben Charles. *The Complete Herbal.* Barre, MA: Barre Publishers, 1972.

Hierbas Mexicanas: Secretos de Curanderos Mexicanos y Plantas Conocidas. Mexico D.F.: Editores Mexicanos Unidos, 1992.

Hispanic Culture and Health Care: Fact, Fiction, Folklore. edited by Ricardo Arguijo Martinez. St. Louis, MO: Mosby, 1978.

Hoffman, David L., *The Herb User's Guide: The Basic Skills of Medical Herbalism.* U.K.: Hazell Watson & Viney Limited, 1987.

Homenaje a Nuestras Curanderas: Honoring Our Healers. Oakland, CA: Latina Press, 1996.

Hudson, William M., editor. *The Healer of Los Olmos and Other Mexican Lore.* Dallas, TX: Southern Methodist Press, 1951.

Kay, Margarita Artschwager. *Healing with Plants in the American-Mexican West.* Tucson, AZ: University of Arizona Press, 1996.

———, John D. Meredith, Wendy Redlinger, and Alicia Quiroz Raymond. *Southwestern Medical Dictionary: Spanish/English, English/Spanish.* Tucson, AZ: University of Arizona Press, 1977.

Kelly, Isabel. *Folk Practices in North Mexico: Birth Customs, Folk Medicine, and Spiritualism in the Laguna Zone.* Austin, TX: University of Texas Press, 1965.

Kiev, Ari., M.D. *Curanderismo: Mexican American Folk Psychiatry.* New York: The Free Press, 1968.

Latorre, Dolores L. *Cooking and Curing with Mexican Herbs: Recipes and Remedies Gathered in Múzquiz, Coahuila.* Austin, TX: Encino Press, 1977.

Leach, Maria, editor. *Funk & Wagnalls Standard Dictionary of Folklore, Mythology, and Legend.* San Francisco: Harper & Row, 1984.

Leung, Albert Y. and Steven Foster. *Encyclopedia of Common Natural Ingredients Used in Food, Drugs, and Cosmetics.* 2nd edition. New York: John Wiley & Sons, Inc., 1996.

Luna, Alvaro *Mil Plantas Medicinales.* Editores Mexicanos Unidos, S.A., 1985.

Lust, John B., N.D., D.B.M. *The Herb Book.* New York: Bantam Books, 1974.

Madsen, Claudia. *A Study of Change in Mexican Folk Medicine.* New Orleans: Middle American Research Institute, Tulane University; 1965.

Martínez, Maximino. *Catalogo de Nombres Vulgares y Científicos de Plantas Mexicanas.* Mexico, D.F.: Fondo de Cultura Económica, 1987.

Medical Botany: Plants Affecting Man's Health. New York: John Wiley & Sons, Inc. 1977.

Meyer, George G., M.D., Kenneth Blum, Ph.D., and John G. Cull, Ph.D., editors. *Folk Medicine and Herbal Healing.* Springfield, IL: Charles C. Thomas, Publisher, Ltd., 1981.

Moore, Michael. *Los Remedios: Traditional Herbal Remedies of the Southwest.* Santa Fe, NM: Red Crane Books, 1990.

———. *Medicinal Plants of the Desert and Canyon West: A Guide to Identifying, Preparing, and Using Traditional Medicinal Plants Found in the Deserts and Canyons of the West and Southwest.* Santa Fe, NM: Museum of New Mexico Press, 1989.

Myer, Michael C. and William L. Sherman. *The Course of Mexican History.* New York: Oxford Universty Press, 1991.

Ody, Penelope. *The Complete Medicinal Herbal.* New York: Dorling Kindersley, Limited, 1993.

Ortiz de Montellano, Bernard. *Aztec Medicine, Health, and Nutrition.* New Brunswick: Rutgers University Press, 1990.

Perez, Jose M. Dichos. *Dicharachos y Refranes Mexicanos.* Mexico, D.F.: Editores Mexicanos Unidos, 1992.

Perrone, Bobette, 1927. *Medicine Women, Curanderas, and Women Doctors.* 1st ed. Norman, OK: University of Oklahoma Press, 1989.

Roeder, Beatrice A. *Chicano Folk Medicine from Los Angeles, California.* Berkeley, Los Angeles, CA: University of California Press, 1988.

Rose, Linda C. *Disease Beliefs in Mexican-American Communities.* San Francisco: R&E Research Associates, 1978.

Rinzler, Carol Ann. *The Complete Book of Herbs, Spices and Condiments: From Garden to Kitchen to Medicine Chest.* New York: Facts on File, 1990.

Schendel, Gordon. *Medicine in Mexico: From Aztec Herbs to Betatrons.* Austin, TX: University of Texas Press, 1968.

Shewell-Cooper, W.E. *Plants, Flowers and Herbs of the Bible: The Living Legacy of the Third Day of Creation.* New Canaan, CT: Keats Publishing, Inc., 1977.

Simon, James E. *Herbs: An Indexed Bibliography: 1971–1980: The Scientific Literature on Selected Herbs and Aromatic and Medicinal Plants of the Temperate Zone.* Amsterdam; New York; Elsevier, 1984.

Spoerke, David G., *Herbal Medications.* Santa Barbara, CA: Woodbridge Press Publishing Company, 1990.

Torres, Eliseo. *Green Medicine: Traditional Mexican-American Herbal Remedies.* Kingsville, TX: Nieves Press.

———. *The Folk Healer: The Mexican-American Tradition of Cruanderismo.* Kingsville, TX: Nieves Press.

Trotter, Robert T., and Juan Antonio Chavira. *Curanderismo: Mexican-American Folk Healing.* Athens, GA: The University of Georgia Press, 1981.

Tylor, Varro E., Ph.D. *The Honest Herbal.* 3rd edition. New York: Hawthorn Press. 1993.

Weiner, Michael A. *The Herbal Bible: A Family Guide to Herbal Home Remedies.* San Rafael, CA: Quantum Books, 1992.

Weiss, Gaea, and Shandor Weiss. *Growing and Using Healing Herbs.* Emmaus, PA: Rodale Press, 1985.

Westrich, LoLo. *California Herbal Remedies.* Houston, TX: Gulf Publishing Co., Book Division, 1989.

Winter, Evelyne. *Mexico's Ancient and Native Remedies.* Mexico, D.F.: Editorial Fournier, S.A., 1968.

Verti, Sebastian. *Tradiciones Mexicanas.* Mexico, D.F.: Editorial Diana, 1994.

Zohary, Michael. *Plants of the Bible: A Complete Handbook to All the Plants with 200 Full-Color Plates Taken in the Natural Habitat.* New York: Cambridge University Press, 1982.